I'm Not Only a Cancer Patient,

I'm a Survivor

A Workbook for Adults

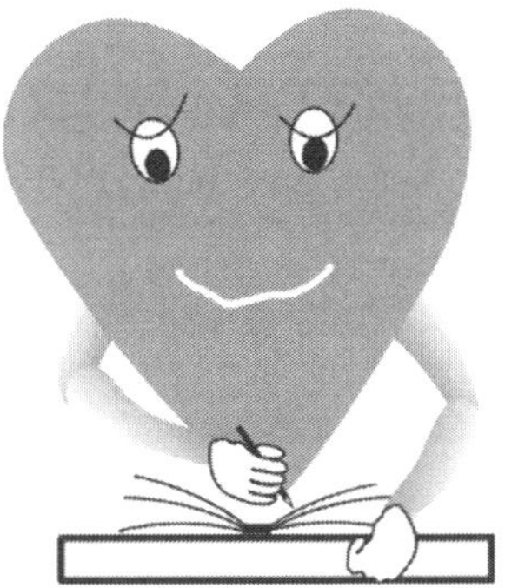

William Penzer Ph.D.

Esperance Press Inc.
150 South University Drive
Plantation FL 33324
954 475 1371
cancerville.com

This book is available at special quantity discounts for bulk purchases, fundraising, educational, or institutional use. Contact media@cancerville.com

ISBN-10: 0983501726

ISBN-13: 9780983501725

Printed in the United States of America

10 9 8 7 6 5 4 3 2 1

Dedication

This Workbook is dedicated to all of the wonderful people I have met in Cancerville— people thriving and striving after surviving.

This includes my wonderful daughter, Jodi, whose Cancerville journey planted the fuse inside my mind for writing *How to Cope Better When Someone You Love Has Cancer*. It also includes Jake who survived his leukemia through sheer will and determination, along with his twin brother Chase's perfect bone marrow match. Their experience lit the fuse that Jodi's planted.

It is dedicated to all of the patients and caregivers (whom I call "heart and soul givers") who have dealt with cancer; all who are dealing with it now; and all who will have to deal with it in the future. I wish you safe passage and Godspeed.

It is also dedicated to the devoted researchers, physicians, and medical teams. It pays tribute to everyone working at cancer centers all over the world. This includes the receptionist at the front desk, the nurses and doctors, the directors of these centers, and everyone in between these important positions.

We are all joined together by a common bond of offering help and hope to those dealing with cancer. Let us continue to work together to make this book, and all others on this topic, obsolete in the near future.

In the meantime, let us continue to extend a strong, warm, and caring hand of support wherever it is needed.

William Penzer, Ph.D.
April 2013

Keep your thoughts positive because your thoughts become your words.

Keep your words positive because your words become your behaviors.

Keep your behaviors positive because your behaviors become your habits.

Keep your habits positive because your habits become your values.

Keep your values positive because your values become your destiny.

—Gandhi

Acknowledgements

My sincere thanks and appreciation to:

My wife, Ronnie, for not only helping me with the edits, but more importantly accepting my work ethic that has allowed me to write three books in less than three years.

My sons, David and Mike, and daughter, Jodi, for always supporting my work in every way they could.

My grandsons, who are growing up to be fine young men. I am confident they will contribute to the world in wonderful ways.

Our miracle granddaughter, who is as beautiful and special as her name.

Bernie Siegel, M.D., who generously took me under his wing and guided my spiritual journey into miracles, blessings, angels, and the like.

My longtime friend and colleague Harvey, a psychologist, author, publisher and business executive, who encouraged me to write this Workbook.

Brad, who has worked on all three book projects, to keep them graphically aligned, and together in ways my computer illiteracy would not allow me to do.

Babs, who designed the cover and the warm heart family characters, intended to symbolize survivorship, love, and taking better care of you.

Justin, who also helped with a variety of technical details.

Good Stuff Monthly, a wonderful little publication, from where many of the quotes were taken.

All of the people who appear in the "Real People Facing Cancer" sections in *How to Cope Better When You Have Cancer,* who taught me so much about strength, courage, dignity, and humility in Cancerville.

All of the unnamed people in South Florida who entrusted me with their minds over all these years, and who taught me so much about how minds work and how to fix them when they don't.

My heartfelt thanks and sincere gratitude goes out to all of you.

With love,

Bill

Preface

In his Foreword to Ari Tuckman's, Psy.D., excellent workbook for ADHD adults, renowned psychiatrist Edward A. Hallowell, M.D., reminisces about how as an elementary school student he hated workbooks:

They were invariably boring. And I hate boring. Workbooks all but defined boring. They always had the drabbest, most unimaginative covers, they were flimsily bound always on the verge of falling apart...

Dr. Hallowell, admittedly had as a youth, and still has, attention deficit disorder, which no doubt guided his career specialization as well as his lack of love for workbooks. Of course, he goes on to praise Dr. Tuckman's workbook as not boring and very helpful, which it is.

Dr. Hallowell's words tripped some switches for me that took me right back to the early grades of school. Though I was not affected by attentional obstacles, I was a most disinterested student until my junior year of college. Dick and Jane were definitely not my friends. I too shuddered and shut down when the teacher said, "Now open your workbooks to page..."

So, my goal in writing and designing this "workbook" was to make it the opposite of boring or anything like the workbooks of my old days at P.S. 64 in the Bronx, New York. Beyond trying to make it interesting, helpful, and stimulating, there is an important difference between this workbook and the ones that distressed Dr. Hallowell, many others, and myself. In this case, you are not obligated to read or participate in every section of the workbook. You are free to pick and choose those sections, which resonate with your needs, participate in those "activities" that will help and support you, and the best part of all—no grades!

In addition, you may wonder why most chapters start with "tion" words. I decided upon that simply because those words are action words. That is exactly the intent of this book. I want to facilitate your taking action every step of your Cancerville way. The more you are in charge and in control, the better you will feel.

Welcome to my "support workbook" companion to *How to Cope Better When You Have Cancer*. I believe you, like many, will find both books very interesting and very helpful. And, both are bound together with a small amount of "crazy" glue to prevent them and you from falling apart, and a large amount of caring, sensitivity, and love to help you through your Cancerville journey.

William Penzer, Ph.D.
January 14, 2013

Table of Contents

PART IV: Helpful Encouragements from which to Draw Strength

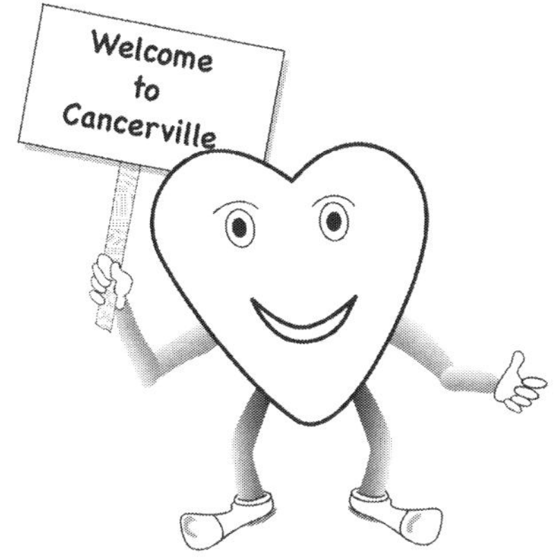

Introduction

So you're cruising down life's highway going as fast as you can, as safely as you can, and doing the best you can. You are studying, and/or working hard, and hopefully playing hard too. You are striving to be a decent person, trying to get ahead, managing your life well, and looking for love in all the right places, and hopefully finding it.

Then, all of a sudden three words completely change your life. It is hard to imagine that is possible—but it is! Instantly, you crash into a brick wall going seventy-miles-per-hour. Someone looks across from you and says, or a voice on the other end of the phone utters these three words: "**You Have Cancer.**" What my friend Susan called a "mortality pie" hits you right in the face, and throws you and your loved ones into a tizzy. All of your priorities shift in a rapid heartbeat. Your focus fixes upon finding medical help and getting answers to a zillion questions racing through your brain like a bullet train.

You have cancer. It's funny how three words can stop you in your tracks and send you to a place of uncertainty and confusion. That was my reality when I was told I had cancer at age 34….I know firsthand that cancer is very scary, but I am living proof that you can survive and thrive after cancer.
—Darren Newberger

In what seems like a microsecond of time, you have entered the place I call Cancerville. Like being in a foreign land, you will find that it has its own culture, customs, language, and technology, amid a variety of confusions and overwhelmtions. It is a place like no other I have been to, which I entered by proxy when my thirty-one-year-old daughter was diagnosed with breast cancer in 2005. She is doing fine and I will share her inspiring story as we go along.

My hope and prayer is that you will do well too. There is no denying that it will take you a while to get the lay of the Cancerville land, and to get past the shock and awful feelings these three words provoke and evoke. Most people find it difficult, initially, to believe that they have cancer. Cancer is what other people get—not you! Acceptance of that most disconcerting idea takes some time. The sooner you accept it, the faster you can move forward—and moving forward is key to your taking charge.

Most important is that you learn to take on Cancerville full tilt. The stronger and more positive you can be, the easier will be your journey—not easy—but easier. For some people I've met, being positive and optimistic comes naturally. They enter Cancerville and ride through it on the horse I call Hope. For others, myself included, it takes much effort and multiple attitude adjustments. It takes a while till we can mount that strong and beautiful horse.

I was raised to be "Chicken Little" by parents obsessed with ever-falling graying skies that quickly turned black. As a result, when our daughter was diagnosed, I was beside myself. This strong, experienced lifeguard on the emotional beach, used to helping people navigate the choppy waters of life, was totally drowning in those very waters.

It took time for me to get a handle on coping in Cancerville, and it took some work too. I used a daily diary, entered counseling, and talked to my self nonstop, like a filibusterer in the Senate. Eventually, I not only learned to cope, but was able to write a book, *How to Cope Better When Someone You Love Has Cancer* to help other "heart and soul givers" do the same. I wrote the book I needed to read that difficult day at Memorial Sloan-Kettering Cancer Center.

It was never my intention to write a book for the cancer patient. However, cancer patients who read the book for the "heart and soul givers" said that it helped them even though they were not the intended audience. They convinced me to write a book for the patient that paralleled the first book. That birthed *How to Cope Better When You Have Cancer.* In preparing to write that book, I spoke to many people who had been to Cancerville. I learned a great deal from them. Here are the common threads of their experiences that they shared. They:

- took charge as best they could
- found ways to feel "in control" given that Cancerville can often feel quite out of control
- were strategic, organized, motivated, and optimistic
- took actions of all kinds
- got back up on the Hope horse quickly, whenever they fell off

This workbook is intended to help you do all of that and more in a structured fashion. It is different in depth and scope from my previous Cancerville books, but it still encourages you to play an active role, and engage in a variety of activities intended to help you manage Cancerville in every way possible. Given that your time is quite limited in Cancerville, this workbook offers you an efficient and effective one-stop place to organize, energize, mobilize, and revitalize your Cancerville journey.

I believe some people will save their workbooks as a record of their experiences, and look back at it periodically. Others, I think, will burn it or throw it away, as another way of putting distance between themselves and Cancerville. I leave that choice to you. Important is that it helps you as you move through Cancerville, and I am very confident that it will. It is undeniable that reading *How to Cope Better When You Have Cancer* and using this workbook, together make for a very empowering support net. Toward that "DAM STRONG!" journey (see Chapter 2), I wish you well.

Your new Cancerville friend,

Bill

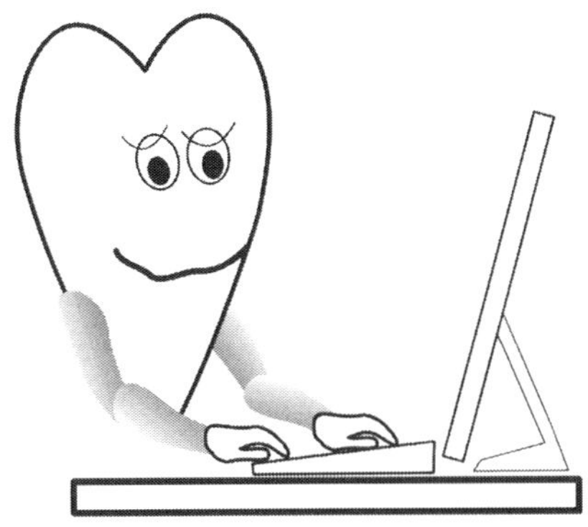

Recommended Resources

In this section I have listed a variety of organizations and their web site addresses that offer helpful information. It is by no means complete, but should allow you to begin to explore the very large universe of Cancerville. These organizations will answer the many questions you have and/or help you find important support.

It is impressive to me that so many helpful organizations exist within the Cancerville community. You are truly not alone, and these organizations truly want to be helpful. And, I've probably missed many, but these should get you off to a good start. If you come across a useful resource that I have missed, please email me at bill@cancerville.com

General Information, Resources, and Support:

- Stupid Cancer…stupidcancer.org
- American Cancer Society…cancer.org
- National Cancer Institute…cancer.gov
- National Coalition for Cancer Survivorship…canceradvocacy.org
- CancerCare…cancercare.org
- CureSearch…curesearch.org
- Lance Armstrong Foundation…livestrong.org
- Cancer Support Community…cancersupportcommunity.org
- ZarpZ…zarpz.org
- Fertile Hope…fertilehope.org
- National Center for Complementary and Alternative Medicine…nccam.nih.gov
- Patient Advocate Foundation…patientadvocate.org
- Coalition of Cancer Cooperative Groups…CancerTrialsHelp.org
- Commission on Cancer…facs.org/cancer/
- Intercultural Cancer Council…iccnetwork.org
- American Pain Foundation…painfoundation.org
- AICR.com
- Integrative Oncology-Essentials.com
- teamfight.org
- robcares.com
- imermanangels.com
- cancerandcareers.org
- CancerHopeNetwork.org
- Cancer.Net
- Caringinfo.org

Children, Teens, and Young Adults

- StupidCancer.org
- Planet Cancer…planetcancer.org
- Ulman Cancer Fund for Young Adults…ulmanfund.org
- mAssKickers.org
- chasingrainbows.ca
- KidsKonnected…kidsconnected.org
- Young Survival Coalition…youngsurvival.org
- Pink Ribbon Girls…pinkribbongirls.org

Blogging:

- caringbridge.org
- carepages.org
- cancerexperienceregistry.org

Transportation/Housing

- Air Charity Network…aircharitynetwork.org
- Corporate Angels Network…CorpAngelNetwork.org
- National Patient Travel Center…PatientTravel.org
- American Cancer Society Hope Lodge…cancer.org/Hope Lodge
- Healthcare Hospitality Network…nahhh.org
- Hospital Hosts…HospitalHosts.com
- Joe's House…JoesHouse.org
- Ronald McDonald House Charities…rmhc.org

Camps and Retreats:

- firstdescents.org
- bluelotusfarm.org
- heartsongretreats.org
- campdream.org

Specific Cancers:

Bone Marrow

- Blood and Bone Marrow Transplant Information Network…BMTinfonet.org
- National Bone Marrow Transplant Link…Nbmlink.org
- National Marrow Donor Program…Marrow.org

Breast

- Young Survival Coalition…youngsurvival.org
- Dr Susan Love Research Foundation…armyofwomen.org
- Force: Facing Our Risk of Cancer Empowered…facingourrisk.org
- Susan G. Komen for the Cure…komen.org
- Annieappleseedproject.org
- Breast Cancer Network of Strength…networkofstrength.org
- Breastcancer.org

- Inflammatory Breast Cancer Research Foundation...ibcresearch.org
- Living Beyond Breast Cancer...lbbc.org
- Sisters Network Inc. ...Sistersnetworkinc.org
- Triple-Negative Breast Cancer Foundation...tnbcfoundation.org

Brain Tumors
- American Brain Tumor Association...abta.org
- The Brain Tumor Foundation...braintumorfoundation.org
- National Brain Tumor Society...braintumor.org

Carcinoid
- The Carcinoid Cancer Foundation...Carcinoid.org
- Caring for Carcinoid Foundation...Caring forCarcinoid.org

Colorectal
- Colon Cancer Alliance...ccalliance.org
- Colorectal Cancer Coalition...fightcolorectalcancer.org
- United Ostomy Associations of America, Inc. ...ostomy.org

Esophageal
- Esophageal Cancer Awareness Association...ECaware.org

Gynecologic
- Gynecologic Cancer Foundation...thegcf.org
- Ovarian Cancer National Alliance...ovariancancer.org
- Foundation for Women's Cancer...FoundationforWomen'sCancer.org
- National Ovarian Cancer Coalition...ovarian.org
- Ovarian Cancer Research Fund...ocrf.org

Head and Neck
- Head and Neck Cancer Alliance...headandneck.org
- Support for People with Oral and Head and Neck Cancer...spohnc.org
- International Association of Laryngectomees...theIAL.org
- The Oral Cancer Foundation...OralCancerFoundation.org

Kidney
- Kidney Cancer Association...kidneycancer.org

Leukemia/Lymphoma/Myeloma
- International Myeloma Foundation...myeloma.org
- Multiple Myeloma Research Foundation...themmrf.org
- The Leukemia and Lymphoma Society...leukemia-lymphoma.org
- National Marrow Donor Program...marrow.org

Liver
- YES...beatlivertumors.org

Lung

- LungCANCER.org
- Lung Cancer Alliance…lungcanceralliance.org
- Lungcancerfoundation.org
- Jillslegacy.org
- LUNGevity Foundation…LUNGgevity.org
- National Lung Cancer Foundation…NationalLungPartnership.org

Mesothelioma

- Pleural Mesothelioma… mesothelioma.org

Myeloma

- International Myeloma Foundation…myeloma.org
- Multiple Myeloma Research Foundation…theMMRF.org

Pancreatic

- Pancreatic Cancer Action Network…pancan.org

Prostate

- Zero—The Project to End Prostate Cancer…zerocancer.org
- Us TOO International, Inc. …Ustoo.org
- Prostate Cancer Foundation…pct.org
- Prostate Cancer Research Institute…prostate-cancer.org

Sarcoma

- Sarcoma Alliance…sarcomaalliance.org
- Sarcoma Foundation of America…curesarcoma.org

Skin

- Melanoma International Foundation…safefromthesun.org
- Skin Cancer Foundation…skincancer.org

Stomach

- Debbie's Dream Foundation: Curing Stomach Cancer…curingstomachcancer.org

Thyroid

- ThyCa: Thyroid Cancer Survivors' Association…thyca.org

Urological

- Bladder Cancer Advocacy Network…bcan.org
- Urology Care Foundation…UrologyHealth.org

PART I

Helpful Ideas from which to Draw Strength

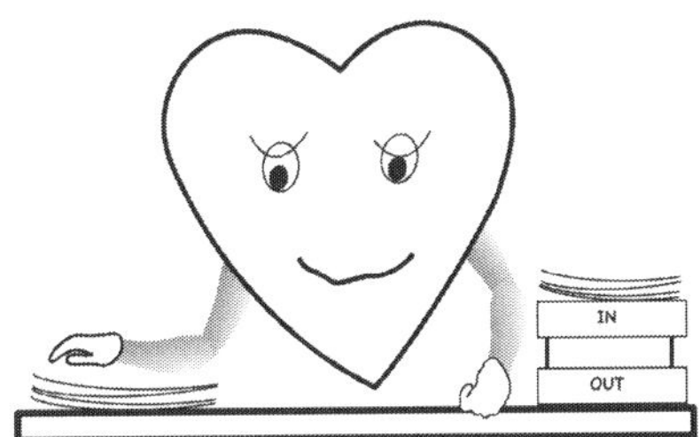

CHAPTER 1

Organization

I debated whether to put this chapter first or last. Remembering that books often linger for a long time on people's nightstands, even though I tried to keep this one short and to the point, I opted to put it first. I hope it will help you get organized for your journey. I understand that you may not be in the mood right now to get organized. That is okay. Feel free to skip it for now, and come back when you are ready to deal with the details.

Dealing with cancer is typically a very overwhelming experience—especially in the beginning. Everything you previously had to do is added to by all that Cancerville demands. In just about all cases, much comes at you much too quickly. The more prepared and better organized you are, the easier will be your journey. In addition, staying organized and being prepared will give you a stronger sense of being in control. As advanced as healthcare is technologically, it can be quite lame when it comes to administrative and insurance details. The more organized you can be the better you will do with that end of this complex multidimensional equation.

If you do not have medical insurance, there are many organizations and governmental agencies to assist. The Patient Advocate Foundation is a really good place to start (patientadvocate.org; 1-800-532-5274). Also try needymeds.org for assistance with medication costs and cassiehinesshoecancer.org for information on travel, financial assistance, and legal resources. This quest may require you putting on your most "assertive shoes," but you can find help. Hopefully, there are people among your "heart and soul giver" team who can help you as well.

The National Coalition for Cancer Survivorship offers a booklet, *What Cancer Survivors Need to Know About Health Insurance*. Here are some of their ideas:

- Read your policy
- Keep good records
- Submit your claims on time and in the right order
- If a claim is denied, appeal it
- Understand your coverage for experimental therapies and clinical trials
- Know where to turn for more information
—canceradvocacy.org

Then again, despite the obstacles, from time to time there is good news:

As reported by Dayve Gabbard, Executive Director of Susan G. Komen South Florida, Florida recently passed an oral chemotherapy parity law. Health insurance companies must now cover the cost of oral cancer drugs in the same way they cover the cost of IV or injectable drugs for all cancer patients in Florida.

The really good news, unrelated to the issues of Cancerville economics, comes from Vincent T. Devita Jr., President of the American Cancer Society Board of Directors. He says, " We can begin to see the end of cancer as a major killer if we continue discovering pathways that attack and prevent cancer or treat it." That is a statement we can all take "to the bank" everyday. It relates to scientists continuing to discover treatments that consist of antibodies specific to the tumor, loaded with anticancer toxin, delivered directly to the site, based upon each patient's genomic data. Though the economic side of Cancerville may be muddled, the growth spurts of its rapidly evolving science are marvelous.

On the practical side, in this chapter you will be able to keep track of appointments, treatments, information gathered, books/websites checked, insurance/billing issues, and so much more. Being organized and having everything in one place helps you feel you have taken charge, reduces the stress of looking for things that were misplaced, and helps the experience flow more smoothly. You need to be the CEO of your Cancerville experience and of yourself. Congrats on being promoted to a job you never wanted, but now have. I am realistically optimistic that you will do your job well.

WEBSITES CHECKED

Address	Focus	Information Learned	Other Sites Suggested

DOCTOR APPOINTMENTS

Doctor	Date	Time	Location	Questions to Ask	Follow-up Appt Date & Time

TREATMENT APPOINTMENTS

Date	Time	Location	Contact	Outp (O)/Inp. (I)	Length of Time	Post-Tx Care	Questions

INSURANCE AND BILLING

Doctor/ Facility	Date of Svc	Amt Billed	Amt Paid by Ins	Amt Owed	Amt Paid/Date Paid	Date of Follow-Up	Contact Person

Doctor/ Facility	Date of Svc	Amt Billed	Amt Paid by Ins	Amt Owed	Amt Paid/Date Paid	Date of Follow-Up	Contact Person

FAMILY AND FRIENDS CONTACTED

Name	Date	Type of Communication (Phone, Email, Other)	Reaction	Follow-up Plan

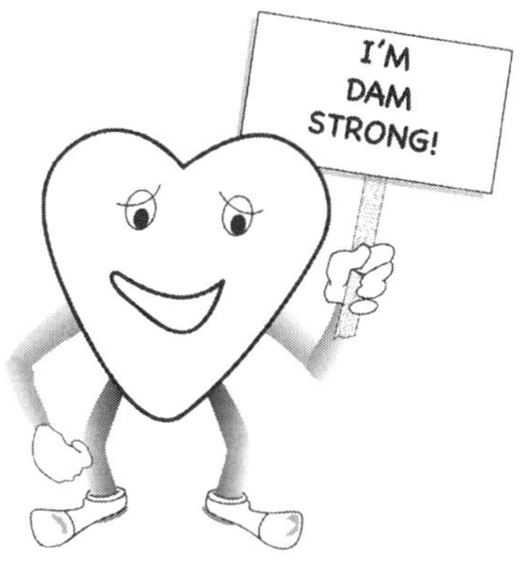

CHAPTER 2

The Origin of "DAM STRONG!"

Though people automatically respond positively to the term "DAM STRONG!" most do not know specifically to what it refers. Since this workbook is devoted to strengthening your Dam in one way or another, let's clarify its meaning right from the beginning. A fuller explanation can be found in Chapter 10 "How Minds Work" in *How to Cope Better When You Have Cancer*, or in Chapter 3 "I Give A Dam" in *Getting Back Up From an Emotional Down*.

In 1973, I shockingly learned that my degree did not come with a vaccine. In a flash, I developed what we now call panic disorder and agoraphobia. Back in the dinosaur days of mental health it was called "neurasthenia"—I kid you not! Back then there were no relevant books, TV talk shows, blogs, Google, etc. There was just five years of suffering through psychoanalysis, flooded with anxiety every step of the way. I kiddingly say I only had one panic attack—it began in '73 and dissipated in '78. That is not as exaggerated as it sounds.

No one could explain to me what had happened to my once seemingly confident self. I went from being a psychologist at IBM, giving presentations to the head honchos, to flipping out when I had to leave the house, or even when the Saturday night babysitter rang the bell to signal I was about to leave my "safe" space. Nor could I easily explain as a new clinician, similar confusions my clients were experiencing (i.e., "Doc. My life is perfect. I have a great wife and kids. No money worries. But I am so depressed I can hardly get out of bed.").

Toward trying to explain myself to myself and understand the people I was helping, I came to believe in certain basic principles that were part of being a person:

- Our histories and all our not so comfortable moments follow us around and can haunt us emotionally. They pop out at the darndest of times.
- Though our minds and bodies are brilliantly constructed, there are some design flaws when it comes to our minds.
- Our brains have storage centers just like computers.
- For simplicity sake, I came up with two storage areas that I called the Cesspool and the Dam.

Success is the culmination of failures, mistakes, false starts, confusion, and the determination to keep going anyway.

—Nick Gleason

There is one thing stronger than all the armies in the world and that is an idea whose time has come.

—Victor Hugo

We either make ourselves miserable or we make ourselves strong. The amount of work is the same.

—Carlos Castaneda

Obstacles are things people see when they take their eyes off the goal.

—Robert Thorpe

Obstacles can't stop you. Problems can't stop you. Most of all, other people can't stop you. Only you can stop you.

—Jeffrey Gilomer

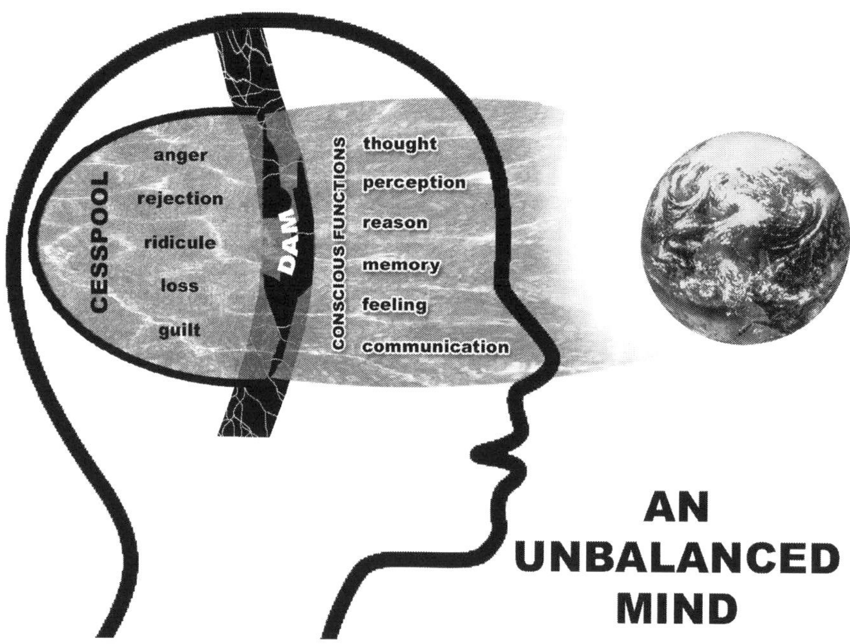

- The Cesspool stores all the negative, hurtful experiences that you encountered from the time you arrived starting with the trauma of birth itself, and concluding with the knowledge that some day you will die. More on the latter later in Chapter 21.
- Every time your feelings were hurt, every time you were chided, every time you "failed" to meet your own goals or those set by others, or felt embarrassed emotional Cess was added to your pool.

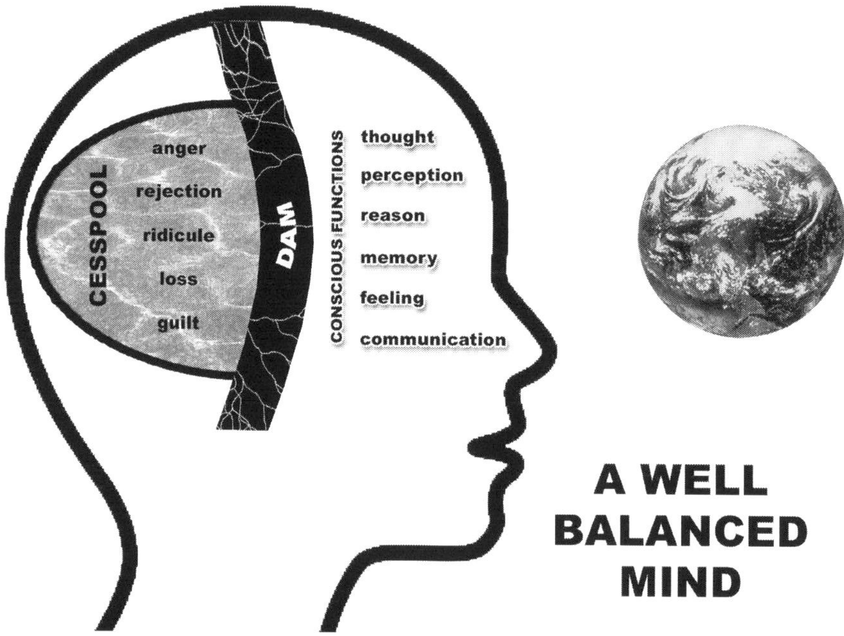

- The Dam stores all of the positive experiences that you encountered from your first kiss, hug, suck of milk on.
- Every time you felt proud, loved, worthy, etc., Dam Grams added to the strength of your Dam.
- As long as your Dam can contain your Cess you feel and function just fine.
- Over time, and in response to a variety of trauma, Dams weaken and Cess intensifies. When that happens anxiety, depression, and a host of other psychological symptoms develop.

- The aim of all therapy, counseling, coaching efforts are to vent Cess and strengthen Dams. When you talk you dump Cess; when I talk I help strengthen your Dam.
- Cess is added by filling your "shame and blame account." Dam grams are added by filling your "pride bank."
- The goal of life is to limit or eliminate "shame and blame" entries and maximize "pride bank" experiences and deposits. The more deposits the stronger your Dam, and the stronger you are to cope with life's challenges.
- The biggest problem with our minds is that they do not have many natural eliminative channels analogous to our body's waste removal systems. Talking and night dreams may be the only direct vents we have.
- Therefore this workbook provides a variety of avenues to vent Cess and strengthen your Dam so you can become "DAM STRONG!"
- Know that you can keep pumping "emotional iron" to counterbalance the Cess of Cancerville, as well as life in general.

Now, more than ever, you need to rise to the challenges of Cancerville and take it on full force. Your Dam needs to be strong and steadfast, and my goal is to help you pump up your mind, even more strongly than it has been before. To be perfectly frank, when my daughter Jodi was diagnosed with breast cancer I fell on my emotional face—"NOT MY KID! NO WAY!!" My Dam collapsed and the old and new Cess poured through like a bucket with a big hole in it. It took me awhile to figure out how to take Cancerville on full tilt and "DAM STRONG!" In writing my books, my only goal was to help you and others get to that point more quickly than I did.

ACTIVITY 1:

Identify the "high tides" of your cesspool.
What are your most sensitive zones?

____

____

____

____

____

If we could take an X-ray of your Cesspool
what do you think we would see?

____

____

____

____

____

People often say that this or that person has not yet found himself. But the self is not something that one finds. It is something one creates.

—Thomas Szasz

When the Dam laughs at the Cesspool, it often comes out in the form of a teardrop.

—William Penzer, Ph.D.
Getting Back Up From an
Emotional Down

Challenges are what make life interesting; overcoming them is what makes life meaningful.

—Unknown

You gain strength, courage, and confidence by every experience in which you really stop to look fear in the face.

—Eleanor Roosevelt

The best way to keep good acts in memory is to refresh them with new ones.

—Raymond Murphy

Better to be a strong person with a weak point, than to be a weak person with a strong point. A diamond with a flaw is more valuable than a brick without a flaw.

—William Boetcker

ACTIVITY 2:

What has helped fill and strengthen your Dam?

________________________________   ________________________________
________________________________   ________________________________
________________________________   ________________________________

Activity: 3

Finish the following sentence with as many words and experiences as you can.
I feel proud that I:

____
____
____
____
____
____

Activity 4:

How has being diagnosed with cancer affected your Cesspool? Has it stirred old fears or added new ones or both?

____
____
____
____

How has being diagnosed with cancer affected your Dam? Is it more or less strong than before your diagnosis?

____
____
____
____

Activity 5:

What actions can you take (i.e., see a mental health professional, talk candidly with friends or family, journal, paint, etc.) that can help you vent Cancerville cess?

____
____
____
____
____

What have you done to strengthen your Dam so far?

____
____
____
____

What can you do from this point on to shore your Dam up even more? If you are not quite sure keep reading!

____
____
____
____

Activity 6:

Here is a place where you can keep track of new cess from Cancerville, so you can focus on venting and neutralizing it. Keep coming back to this page

____
____
____
____
____
____
____

Here is a place you can keep track of ways you have added Dam grams to help support you. Keep coming back to this page.

____
____
____
____
____
____
____
____
____
____

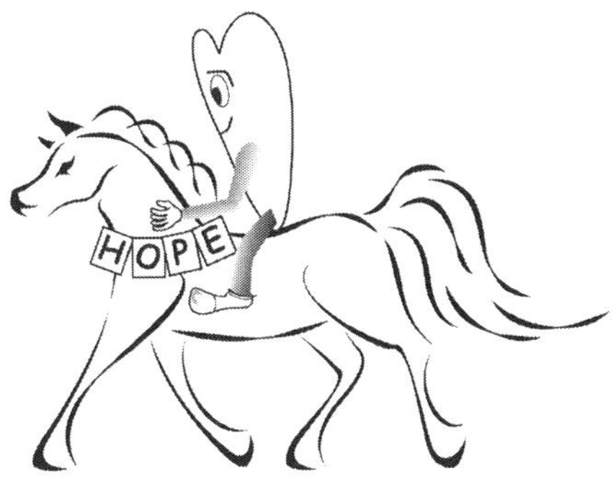

CHAPTER 3

The Ingredients of Hope

Last May, I was invited to The Weekend of Hope in Stowe, Vermont. Every year for the past twelve, the city of Stowe invites cancer patients and their "heart and soul givers" to come to a weekend support conference. The town provides complimentary rooms to over three hundred people.

I was given the honor of being the opening speaker on Friday night. I decided to talk to the audience about what I believed were the ingredients of Hope. These were:

- laughter
- relaxed feelings
- connections with love
- empowerment
- spirituality

For the first, I told a joke or two and had the audience laughing. Laughter is an important healing force and I encourage you to seek it out in any way you can. I understand Cancerville is not a laughing matter, but laughter matters there as in other stressful places. Once the audience was laughing I said, "We are laughing in Cancerville. Let's keep doing that! When we laugh at the enemy we diminish its power."

> *I think part of what made me a comedy writer is the blocking out of some of the really ugly stuff— painful things in my childhood—and covering it up with a humorous attitude…do something to laugh until I was able to forget what was hurting.*
> *—Neil Simon*
> *Playwright*

Most of the important things in the world have been accomplished by people who have kept on trying when there seemed to be no hope at all.

—Dale Carnegie

Finding temporary and specific causes for misfortune is the art of hope.

—Martin Seligman, Ph.D.

I didn't really find anything about cancer funny, but I discovered that funny things continued to exist.

—Evan Handler
Actor

Humor gives us smiles, laughter and gaiety. Humor reveals the roses and hides the thorns. Humor makes our heavy burdens light and smoothes the rough spots in our pathways.

—Sam Ervin

Laughter is a tranquilizer with no side effects.

—Unknown

There's nothing like humor to burst what seems to be an enormous problem.

—Jean Stapleton
(aka Edith Bunker)

Pessimism never won any battles.

—Dwight David Eisenhower

The rarest courage is the courage of thought.

—Unknown

Our prayers are answered not when we are given what we ask, but when we are challenged to be what we can be.

—Morris Adler

Don't rush to change your general approach to coping with cancer. Good attitudes and good access to support including groups can help.

—Jimmie C. Holland, M.D., and
Sheldon Lewis
Authors, The Human Side of Cancer

> *When we laugh, we take our eyes off ourselves and our problems, even if only for a brief moment. It's in that brief moment that we are freed of our daily worries, that we become lightened—in mood and in spirit. And, like a great helium balloon, we rise up and float above the concerns of our world below…. Laughter empowers the human heart to fly.*
> —Rev. Susan Sparks
>   High Places of the Heart
>   Coping with Cancer Magazine

Then I had the group do a brief progressive relaxation exercise. An Omm-like hush filled the ballroom as the audience became more and more relaxed. I encourage you to do relaxation every day. We will talk more about that in Chapters 15 and 16.

Next, I had them all stand and hold hands so we all formed one large circle of connection. I asked them to think of brief loving message in their heads, allow it to come down their left arm and out their hearts. I encouraged that the messages of loving connection would flow all around the room and it would take, according to my calculations, thirty-six seconds to go around. To my delight everyone participated and the smiles on their faces told the tale. We will talk more about the importance of being connected with love and support in Chapter 10.

> *A strong-minded local politician was diagnosed with colon cancer at age fifty. She immediately became a strong advocate of colonoscopies at age forty, as her doctor told her the tumor was likely growing for ten years. Here's what she had to say about her situation and her hopefulness:*
>
> *I plan on fighting this with tremendous dignity and courage…. Having cancer is nothing to be embarrassed about. There is nothing you did to get cancer…. I am going to be OK. I know I am.*
> —Sheila Alu

I then asked them to remain standing, no longer holding hands, and join the chorus of the song I played—Elton John's, "I'm Still Standing." Though it was originally intended to address a former lover, it fits Cancerville just as well. The audience screamed and squealed out the "I'm Still Standing" line! They were all relaxed, connected, and became more empowered. This workbook aims to guide you in those same directions.

Finally, I played "Hallowed Ground," a song from Barbra Streisand's album of the same name. I asked them to interpret it any way they choose, while finding healing spiritual images consistent with their beliefs. I specified this was not so much about religious beliefs, but their higher power supports.

As this song concluded, everyone in the room had experienced my five ingredients of Hope and we knew we were standing on hallowed ground—made that way by previous participants from years past. We will discuss this important topic in Chapter 20, based upon what Bernie Siegel, M.D., taught me about miracles, blessings, angels, and the like.

I am sure there are many other ingredients to Hope as well, and we shall explore all of them in the pages that follow. I am convinced that when we approach any challenging situation hopefully, not only does it improve our chances of being successful, but it makes the journey a little easier and more comfortable. I hope you do or will come to agree with me. I hope to return to Stowe for this marvelous weekend every year, and recently attended and presented at their 2013 weekend.

So, my assignment for this chapter is simple. Laugh a lot; Get a little more relaxed (see Chapters 15 and 16); connect with people you love, even if it is by phone or email (see Chapter 10); begin to feel a small surge of empowerment; and start to get in touch with your spiritual parts (see Chapter 20). Even people who are not religious have spiritual parts that need to be dusted off, experienced, and followed, as they offer healing salves for wounded minds and bodies.

My goal is that by the time you reach the end of this Workbook, you will be riding through Cancerville on the horse I call Hope with the skill, strength, and agility of a cowpoke!

> *It was a long process, but the day my hope was first fed is the day I began to get well. I learned that the heart and the mind must first seek and believe in health in order for the body to find it.*
> *—Vickie Girard*
>   *Author, There's No Place Like Hope*

Beauty triumphs over suffering in heaven and in life.

—Nietzsche

Difficulty is the nurse of greatness.

—William Cullen Bryant

Attitude is the mind's paintbrush— it can color any situation.

—Loring Forcier

We must accept finite disappointment but we must never lose hope.

—Martin Luther King Jr.

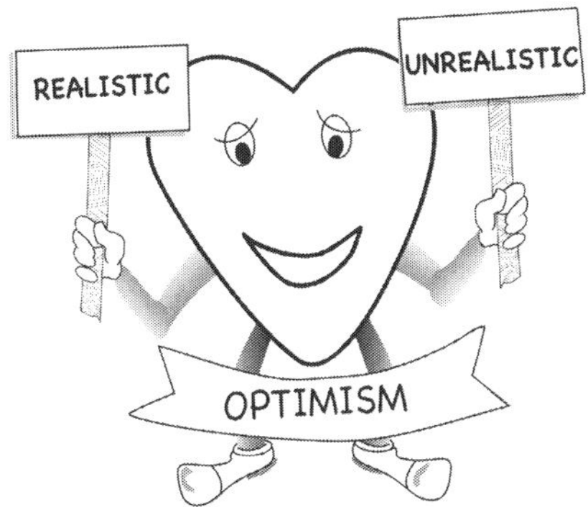

CHAPTER 4

Realistic and Unrealistic Optimism

Realistic Optimism

I called the philosophy that evolved from my Cancerville-by-proxy experience realistic optimism. It reflects the simple-minded idea that if it is realistic, you need to push yourself toward being optimistic. It took me a while to get there. Cancerville intimidated me like no place I have ever been.

The odds we were given by the Sloan-Kettering doctors were always well in Jodi's favor. It took me a while though, to embrace them as part of a realistic optimistic way of thinking. We "Chicken Littles" of the world do not easily embrace or believe in positive outcomes. As we will see, we can learn how to process our experiences differently and become more optimistic.

Bob's ninety percent survival rate for sinus cancer bodes well for his future. To me, it is realistic for him to be optimistic and sustain hope in being able to watch his granddaughter grow up. Truth be known, life is life-threatening, but we have various denial mechanisms to ignore thinking or worrying about all the different paths to Heaven in addition to cancer. Best you try to see cancer as another challenging, but non-lethal experience, unless you have been given information to the contrary. Then it is time to go to unrealistic optimism, while making peace with your fate.

None of the above is intended to downplay the seriousness of cancer, any other major medical problem, or the byproducts of medical treatments. Bob endured very painful surgery and thirty rounds of radiation five days a week. He is still dealing with fatigue, a slowly recovering sense of smell and taste, as well as a tingling sensitivity in his right cheek and an ever-present sniffle. I never said having cancer was easy. I do, however, believe that following a realistic optimistic set of beliefs makes the Cancerville journey a little easier. In fact, I am realistically optimistic that this workbook will help your journey to be a little more comfortable.

Unrealistic Optimism

Well after Jodi and our family distanced ourselves from Cancerville, this not so young student met up with a slightly older hero—Bernie Siegel, M.D. I sat in his backyard for one-and-a-half hours while he talked to me about miracles, angels, blessings, and the like. I had read *Love, Medicine &*

The pessimist complains about the wind; the optimist expects it to change; the realist adjusts the sails.

—William Ward

Beating breast cancer reinforced my ability to live for today and be positive for the future. Keep your sunny side up, keep yourself beautiful, and indulge yourself. I hoped my positive attitude could help someone else going through it.

—Betsy Johnson
Fashion Icon

If you see the glass as half-empty, I can't convince you it is half-full. It is not easy to change people's ingrained attitudes and patterns of coping.

—Jimmie C. Holland, M.D., and
Sheldon Lewis Authors,
The Human Side of Cancer

The difference between a successful person and others is not a lack of strength, not a lack of knowledge, but rather a lack of will.

—Vince Lombardi

Where there is great love there are always miracles.

—Unknown

Forgiving means to pardon the unpardonable; Faith means believing in the unbelievable; and Hoping means to hope when things are hopeless.

—GK Chesterton

We couldn't conceive of a miracle if none had ever happened.

—Libbie Fudim

If someone tells you that you have a three percent chance of surviving cancer, assume you will be in the three percent club!

—Jerry Kaplan
Two time cancer survivor

Miracles when it first came out in the '80s, but my semi-scientific mind was never able to embrace the "miracle" part with all its invisible forces. He helped me cross the bridge that I had already begun to walk on.

> *Accepting that there are forces at work in the universe beyond those under my control required a certain amount of letting go….I had many experiences where I felt I had encountered angels on earth, but now I was open to a new world of communication with the angels above.*
> *—Beth DuPree, M.D.*
> *Author, The Healing Consciousness*

Over the years, those forces became more and more evident to me. Years ago I concluded, "There are no coincidences in life, just endless opportunities and possibilities." It was that belief that led me to have the courage to contact Bernie in the first place, which has led to a pleasant relationship and easy communication. Bernie's discourse that day, jam-packed with examples from his years as a surgeon as well as his personal life, helped me to realize the blessings, miracles, and angels that have been part of my life too.

As I sat there in the sunshine listening to Bernie, I came to realize that we have all experienced the powerful influence of invisible forces lurking about that lacked rhyme or reason. Whether we call them God's work, blessings, a lucky punch, miracles, or a meant to be experience doesn't really matter. That these hard to explain, but influential potentials are all around us is hard to deny.

In this context I am encouraging you, at certain times, to indulge in unrealistic optimism. Even when the odds are against you, try your hardest to believe that a miracle can come along and overturn those odds.

> *Jake and Chase, the twins whose story stimulated my writing "How to Cope Better When Someone You Love Has Cancer" faced long odds and physician pessimism in overcoming Jake's Leukemia. Jake is alive and well today thanks to the doctor's fine work despite the odds, and his brothers perfect and miraculous bone marrow match.*
>
> *I am convinced the prayer groups Rob organized all over the world helped too. On a specific day at a specific time, wherever we were in the world we were to send Jake healing prayers. Ronnie and I once set the clock for the middle of the night when traveling in Australia.*
>
> *A few weeks ago, this eleven-year-old boy had his dream fulfilled by skating out onto center ice with his heroes, the New York Rangers. Now that my friends, is a miracle and a blessing that came straight from the thousands of prayers chanted by us all in Jake's name.*

Obviously, if you face long odds it is time to get your house in order. This will be discussed in more detail in Chapter 21. However, while doing that leave room for a Hail Mary pass or whatever that may be unrealistic, but still possible. In that vein, I am sending a fair amount of fairy dust in your direction. Bernie's more recent books, *A Book of Miracles* and *faith, hope & healing* offer many examples of people who were told to prepare for their trip to heaven, who are still here on earth. As the sign in my office says, "NEVER, NEVER, NEVER GIVE UP!"

> *Miracles are not spontaneous remissions—they are cases of self-induced healing. The more we learn about healing, and open ourselves up to it happening, the more likely they are to occur.*
> *—Bernie Siegel, M.D.*
> *Personal Communication*

Let us also remember that no one, not even Cancerville doctors, have a crystal ball—no one can predict the future with certainty. Doctors have the results of large research studies from which their numbers come. That may or may not relate to your unique situation, so please take all feedback, good or not so good, with a grain of salt. My physician friend Bob, many years ago said, "Bill, in any medical situation the odds are either 100% or 0% of people surviving. All the rest is a guess!" For now, assume that your odds of becoming a survivor are 100%!

> *To me, miracles are about our potential and what has been built into us to help us to survive.*
>
> *—Bernie Siegel, M.D.*
> *A Book of Miracles*

> *No matter how bad things are they can always be worse. So what if my stroke left me with a speech impediment? Moses had one, and he did all right.*
>
> *—Kirk Douglas*

PART II

Helpful Fuel from which to Draw Strength

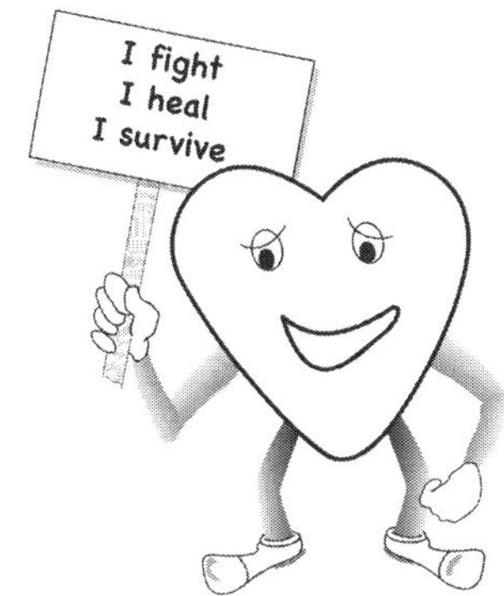

CHAPTER 5

Motivation

Survival is one powerful motivator! Much as we know we are all going to die someday, none of us want to anytime soon. "Someday" is the operative word in the last sentence. Bernie Siegel, M.D., in discussing our mortality in his immortal book *Love, Medicine & Miracles* said, "No one lives forever; therefore death is not the issue. Life is. Death is not a failure. Not choosing to take on the challenges of life is." Throughout this workbook I am encouraging, nudging, and at times, pushing you to take on the challenges of Cancerville. At the end of the day that is really all you can do!

> *No one will tell you that cancer is going to be easy, There will be times when you feel like you just can't get locked into the radiation mask one more time, or like you can't muster up the strength to even get hooked up to that chemo IV. But you have to. Like a cute little furry badger, when times get tough and your very existence is threatened, it's time to "badger up" and fight like you've never fought before.*
> *—Glenn Brooks*
> *Survivor*
> *Coping with Cancer Magazine*

The question arises as to what being motivated means in the context of having cancer and how one strengthens that motivation to be at the ready for Cancerville? Think of a professional athlete on the field of play, a soldier on the front lines of battle, or a proud parent taking care of a newborn. All share similar characteristics:

Being

- focused and alert
- attentive to details
- single-minded
- dedicated and committed to their goals
- calm and patient
- energized

When something bad happens you have three choices. You can either let it define you, let it destroy you, or let it strengthen you.

—Unknown

Crises redefine life. In them you discover what you are.

—Allan Knight Chalmers

Bravery is the capacity to perform properly even when scared half to death.

—Gen. Omar Bradley

You have brains in your head.
You have feet in your shoes.
You can steer yourself
Any direction you choose.

—Dr. Seuss

This is how I would want you to be as you take on Cancerville full tilt. The exercises that follow are aimed at pumping you up for game day, getting you psyched and ready to do battle, and healing yourself with nourishing, nurturing self-love.

Much as some do not like warrior words, I view Cancerville as a battle royal, not much different than the battlefields of Iraq, or Afghanistan. For that reason I want you prepared, trained and armed, ever ready to take it on head-on. In this David and Goliath battle your mind and self-talk are your slingshot. Please remember who won that lopsided battle.

> *You see I did get a war—just not the one I expected. Rather, my war turned out to be one against an unseen enemy that I've battled for many years now. It's a war that still goes on today, and one that short of a miracle, I expect to fight for the rest of my life.*
> *—Jay Platt*
> *Retired Marine*
> *Survivor von Hippel Laindau Syndrome*
> *Author, No Matter What*

Let's assume, that like David, you too will win your battle and become a survivor. In fact, like my tee shirt and the title of this book says, you are one already. And, tough as warriors may be when they have to be, they are quick to take R&R when they can. I just want you growling when you need to face surgery, chemo, or radiation. GRRR! I want you meditating when you are healing. OMMM!

Activity 1:

Please think of a time or two when you had to get your "game" going (i.e., big test, taking your driver's test, job interview, presentation, customer call, wedding, giving birth, car accident with you injured, surgery, etc. Please list all the ways you pumped up for this demanding event:

____

____

____

____

____

____

Activity 2:

Did you do anything differently for one challenge than you did for another? If yes please list those below. For example, for tests, presentations, oral defense of my Ph.D. and the like I tended to over-prepare.

The only way for me to fight cancer was like a vicious pit bull.

—Terry Crowley
Bladder Cancer Survivor

You can't be a smart cookie if you have a crummy attitude.

—Unknown

The difference between try and triumph is just a little umph!

—Martin Phillips

Fate cannot be changed; otherwise it would not be fate. Man, however, may well change himself, otherwise he would not be man.

—Victor Frankel

When people are highly motivated, it's easy to accomplish the impossible And when they're not, it's impossible to accomplish the easy.

—Bob Collings

For my wedding, I talked to myself in my voice of reassurance. For medical situations, I did both of those and also assumed I would be fine and that my doctors knew what they were doing. When my mind went tilt I read, sought professional help, went to the gym, and did whatever I could to strengthen my Dam.

The more you can identify the ingredients to your "pumping up" under past challenging conditions, the more you can draw from them right now. We all cope differently, draw from different skill sets, and depend upon different tools and activities. How you cope better is your choice. That you cope as well as you possibly can is essential.

____
____
____
____
____
____
____
____
____

Activity 3:

Using these past energizing motivators, what kind of an emotional "cocktail" can you whip up to whip yourself into shape?

I can do the following to get myself psyched and ready for dealing with the demands and challenges of Cancerville:

____
____
____
____
____

Activity 4:

Write down how you will know that you are motivated, pumped and "DAM STRONG!"
I will know because I will *feel as strong as a Sumo wrestler.*
I will know because I will *feel at peace within myself.*
I will know because I will *feel* ____
I will know because I will *feel* ____
I will know because I will *feel* ____
I will know because I will think *more positively.*
I will know because I will think ____
I will know because I will think ____
I will know because I will think ____
I will know because I will think ____

Activity 5:

What resources can you draw upon to add to your strength and motivation? Examples include family and friends, people who have dealt with cancer, partner, inspiring books, religion, counselor/coach, support groups, blogs, web sites, etc. Please write down all of your sources and resources that will help you take on Cancerville.

_____*Read: How to Cope Better When You Have Cancer.*
_____*Read any helpful and inspiring book cited in this Workbook that appeals to you.*

____
____
____
____
____

Activity 6:

On a scale of 1-10 where 10 is "Dam Strong!" circle the number where you feel you are at right now when it comes to energy, motivation, and power:

1   2   3   4   5   6   7   8   9   10

Are you comfortable with that level?   Circle one: Yes   No

If No, what else can you do to pump up?

____
____
____
____
____

Activity 7:

As your strength wanes or grows please come back to this scale for updates and revised plans. Keeping yourself pumped through your Cancerville journey is an important piece of the puzzle.

0   1   2   3   4   5   6   7   8   9   10

____
____
____

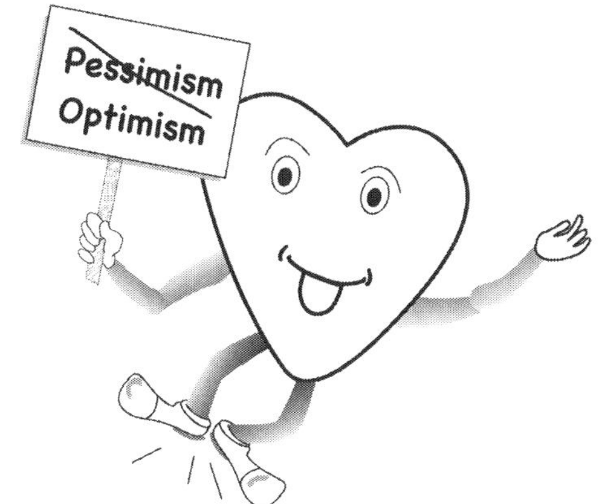

CHAPTER 6

Optimization

For me, the best way to optimize outcomes in life is to be optimistic about them and take actions consistent with that perspective. The more hopeful and positive we are, the more likely the results will be optimized. It almost doesn't matter what the event happens to be. It could be a test you are taking, a speech you are giving, a dinner party you are making, or a medical procedure your team is doing. Research has consistently demonstrated that optimistic expectations lead to positive results—over and over again.

> *There's this big C looming over us, pressing us under its weight, threatening to dominate our daily lives for the next however-long. But stop. Take a breath. Tell yourself you have to be positive, because you're the one in the driver's seat here. You may have to work at it a little, and the change may not take place overnight. Being positive can take practice. More than anyone else, though, you can make it happen.*
> —Barbara Delinsky
> Breast Cancer Survivor and Author

Self-fulfilling prophecy is alive and doing very well in all of us. Though it does not necessarily work for games of chance, lotto, or other events unrelated to our mindly influence, it does work when how and what we think can effect both the process and the outcome. Think of a speech, job interview, or presentation. If we are negative about our performance potentials we will be more anxious and self-conscious. This, in turn, will affect how we do as we will be limited and distracted by those intrusions. On the other hand, if you are calm, comfortable, and confident you will fly high on your own power, and on the wings of angels who rally to positive people.

As for medical issues the data is clear and consistent. Expect negative happenings in the form of pain, scarring, fatigue, terrible side effects, and the like and the likelihood is you will get just that. Expect the opposite and the likelihood is you will get just that.

As you already know, the mind and the body are so interwoven and interactive in their connections that you have much mental power to tap

Life's battles don't always go to the strongest or fastest—sooner or later those who win are those who think they can.

—Richard Bach

I do not feel any less of a woman. I made a strong choice that no way diminishes my femininity.

—Angelina Jolie

Good thoughts bear good fruit, bad thoughts bear bad fruit— and man is his own gardener.

—James Allen

Of all the forces that make for a better world, none is so indispensable, none so powerful as hope. Without hope man is only half-alive.

—Charles Sawyer

Life inflicts the same setbacks and tragedies on the optimist as on the pessimist, but the optimist weathers them better… Even when things go well for the pessimist he is haunted by forebodings of catastrophe.

—Martin Seligman, Ph.D.

I chose to never give up, to fill my heart with love, to take control of the new journey I found myself on, and to embrace every day….I embrace life on a new level…with courage and faith.

—Lynda Peterson

A strong positive mental attitude will create more miracles than any wonder drug.

—Patricia Neal

into. Not only does that power help to influence the process, it also helps you feel more comfortable and confident as you go through your Cancerville experience. This is precisely why I said earlier that your mind is your slingshot in this David and Goliath battle.

Having hopeful feelings also preps you to be better able to deal with the stresses of the day. Though every professional in Cancerville is on your side and rooting for you, some days it may not feel that way. This occurs when you wait hours for an appointment, a receptionist is having a bad "head" day, or your doctor rushes you out the door before you have asked half your questions. These are times when your optimism, hopefulness, and trust need to be at their strongest and most empowering levels.

In his research on optimism and on how to teach pessimistic people to become more optimistic, Dr. Seligman identified some differences between optimists and pessimists. These differences relate to one's "explanatory style"—the way in which you typically explain why events happen.

Pessimist	Optimist
See negative events as permanent.	See negative events as temporary.
See negative events as all encroaching (i.e., Bob said to himself, " I have cancer. My life is ruined. Nothing will be okay ever again.")	See negative events as specific to that area (i.e., Susan said "I have cancer, I am NOT cancer."
Blame themselves for negative events.	Blame external forces for negative events.

My strong encouragement is that you be a strong encourager for yourself to optimize your resources, strength, comfort, and hopefully success in your survivorship. All of you—your body, mind, and spirit—need to be in sync by anticipating positive outcomes, over and over again.

Being down, distressed, or debilitated is par for the Cancerville course. Staying that way is unhealthy for mind, body, and spirit. When you can, pick yourself up, dust yourself off, and look for inspiring supports and energizing encouragements. Life, in all ways, can be quite a challenge. Cancerville is one of the most challenging arenas that we can enter. Who better than you to take it on?

Yoko Ono, John Lennon's widow, was asked to explain why the Beatle's were such an incredible phenomenon in their day. As she gazed out over the Strawberry Fields memorial to their music in Central Park she said, "I think they had so much hope. We all had such hope then. And when you have that kind of hope, you can accomplish anything."

Optimism…is not a panacea. But it can protect you against depression; it can raise your level of achievement; it can enhance your physical well being; it is a far more pleasant mental state to be in.
—Martin Seligman, Ph.D.

Everyone has a burden; what counts is how you carry it.
—Joe Brown

When the going gets tough, the tough get going.
—Unknown

There are some professionals who worry that encouraging optimism and positive attitudes put pressure on the patient. He or she may feel like they are failing when they have trouble sustaining those feelings. First, there is no such thing as failing in Cancerville. However you do it, is your way and right for you. Second, I acknowledge repeatedly, that most fall off the horse I call Hope from time to time, just as I did.

I do encourage that you try to scramble back up when you can. Finally, I agree totally with Dr. Seligman. Our belief is that independent of the outcome, being hopeful makes the journey a little more tolerable and a little more comfortable. Clearly, as a psychologist, I want you to be open and honest with your feelings, especially during the rough patches. It is not about hiding from deep-seated feelings or pretending hope when it is not there. It is about seeking hope out when you can and making it part of your Cancerville mantra.

When you focus solely on the positive, it shuts down the patient's ability to confide in you about a fear of the future or the negative emotions they might have.
—Hoda Badr, Ph.D.

Clear your mind of can't.
—Solon

According to Cure's Cancer Resource Guide, 2010:

As you begin to tell others about your diagnosis, you may feel pressure to maintain a positive attitude, which can be especially difficult when you are scared, anxious, or not feeling well. False optimism is unrealistic, and experts say feeling you are not "doing cancer right" can be a huge burden.

Activity 1:

Do you consider yourself a pessimist, optimist, or combo? (circle one)
Write down some examples that demonstrate your answer?

____

____

____

____

____

____

Activity 2:

If you tend toward pessimism or selective combo pessimism/optimism are you willing to try your best to shift closer to a more positive perspective? Yes   No   Maybe (circle one)

If No, I respect your right to be whom you need to be as you continue your Cancerville journey.

If Maybe, may I nudge you toward YES?

If Yes, nice!

Activity 3:

If Yes, GO for it the Nike way and "Just Do It!" or use my "Push Your Tush" mantra to move back toward hopeful feelings. Please write down at least eight things you can do to raise the bar toward a more positive, optimistic, and hopeful approach. I will give you the first four, but you owe me—actually you owe you—four more:

1) *Read Dr. Seligman's book "Learned Optimism."*
2) *Ride through Cancerville on a horse I call Hope!*
3) *Give yourself permission to fall off her from time to time.*
4) *Use Affirmations every day. See Chapter 8.*
5) ____
6) ____
7) ____
8) ____

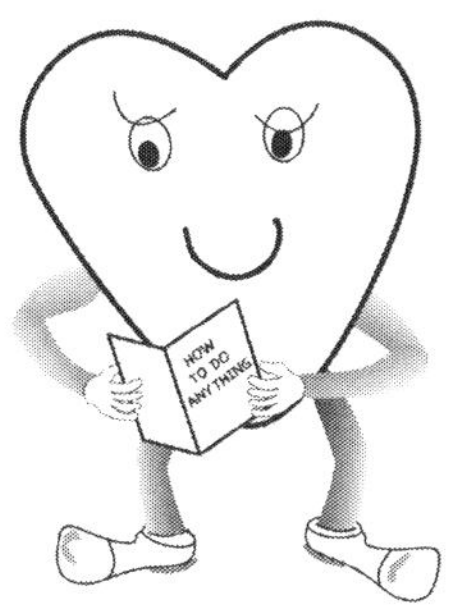

CHAPTER 7

Adaptation

In a dazzling display of innate human potential, we splendidly adapt to our environs. When they are pleasant, such as a party or vacation, we enjoy the positive experiences, but still need to adapt in a variety of ways. When my wife and I go on a cruise we have to adapt to downsizing from the comfortable space of our home, to the doll-house-like size of our cabin. None-the-less we have fun and relax—at least to the extent the robot within me allows!

Obviously, cancer is no cruise or cakewalk! It is a difficult and demanding place that challenges you at every turn. The word itself brings chills to your spine, and back in the day, the word was never uttered except perhaps in hushed tones or referred to as the big C. This is what made Time Magazine's headline of April 1, 2013 a little too in my face—"How to Cure Cancer."

Though the title was a little too matter of factly presented (almost like an April fools dark joke), and sounded a little too "slam dunkish" for me, the article itself was excellent. It described how different medical teams are now working together for the good of the cause. They are adapting to the needs of Cancerville to move forward more rapidly. This movement is being sponsored and supported by the entertainment industry through a group they formed called Stand Up 2 Cancer (SU2C). The metaphor they are using is that cancer research needs to flow the way Hollywood makes movies, drawing from a large pool of talent all working together in a "time is of the essence" fashion.

Just as the scientific community is adapting to advancing cancer technology, so you will need to adapt to dealing with Cancerville. Once you get past the shock and awful, or perhaps even before you completely do, you will need a tactical plan through which to confront and navigate your journey. If Cancerville is a war zone, then you will need to arm yourself with the right ammunition to survive. In my way of thinking, first you fight back with all your might, and then you take time to heal with all the bright light you can muster.

From my book *How to Cope Better When You Have Cancer* comes these words:

Catastrophes and crises create chaos, which in turn demands immediate adjustment. Entering Cancerville is obviously a crisis of grand proportion, but one that you will manage. As people we adapt naturally and automatically to life's demands. Think of times in the

The harder I worked, the smarter I became. The smarter I became the more mindful I remained. The more mindful I remained, the luckier I got.

—*George P. Kansas*
Survivor
Author, iCanSir!

How a person masters his fate is more important than what his fate is.

—*Wilhelm Von-Humboldt*

Intentions may be written in pencil; commitments should be carved in stone.

—*Robert Thorpe*

It is easy to sit up and take notice. What is difficult is getting up and taking action.

—*Thomas Fuller*

We have to learn to be our own best friends, because we fall too easily into the trap of being our worst enemies.

—Roderick Thorp

Though I personally experienced a full range of negative feelings as I entered Cancerville as a "heart and soul giver," I came to realize that those feelings were hurtful and toxic to my family and myself.

—William Penzer, Ph.D.

Facts that are not frankly faced have a habit of stabbing us in the back.

—Harold Bowden

Pain nourishes courage. You can't be brave if you've only had wonderful things happen to you.

—W.B. Prescott

Swing hard, in case they throw the ball where you're swinging.

—Duke Snider

> *past when you had to cope with and adjust to difficult situations. Reminding yourself how you were able to do it then will help you gain confidence that you can do it again now.*
> *—William Penzer, Ph.D.*

The computer has made adaptation in general, and particularly in Cancerville, much easier. People vary in their need for knowledge ranging from burning the midnight oils searching for information, to minimal interest beyond the basics. I warn you that, for some people, that search can become addictive and that, as you know, not all information on the Internet is accurate. Watch out for those lurking in the shadows looking to take advantage of fearful and vulnerable people for financial gain and your loss.

In addition to gaining knowledge and information, many of the sites listed in the Resource section will help you find a variety of support nets that offer help and hope.

> *The most powerful tool to guide you in your journey through cancer is knowledge. Learning about your condition can give you confidence, comfort, and help you feel more in control.… Your physician and other members of your health care team can supply you with trustworthy information and resources.*
> *Caring4Cancer*

Practical matters will guide your adaptation. Where you live, your medical insurance, your support network, whether you have children, the type of work you do, your financial resources, and a host of many other factors will lead you to make decisions and choices that fit for you. The last two words of the last sentence are very important. Remember this is your journey and you are the leader of the pack and top dog. Everyone else needs to follow and support your lead—at least if you are making self-protective choices. Others who love you do have the right to offer opinions if they feel you are not taking the most self-protective path. We had to arm-wrestle Jodi post-surgery into going through with chemo as she did not want to for obvious reasons. The doctors called it "insurance." I called it survivorship.

> *There were times I felt like my body had turned against me. I couldn't eat; I couldn't sleep; I had no energy. It was probably the worst experience of my life, but on the flip side, I knew this was a process that had the ability to cure me of lymphoma forever. So I had to trust in the process.*
> *—Ethan Zohn*
> * Africa Survivor Winner*

There are many tools of adaptation beyond information gathering and decision-making. The first is acceptance, which does take some time to embrace. Ultimately, most people accept that they have been dealt a difficult hand, and rise accordingly to its challenges.

Of course, perseverance is important. You will need to keep it firmly in place for the duration. The twists and turns in Cancerville can be overwhelming, as can be the confusions, miscommunications, detours, and changes in treatment direction. Perseverance allows you to just keep pushing forward no matter the obstacles until you get past them as a survivor.

Madam Curie identifies the next adaptive characteristic by mentioning confidence. Once a plan has been set in motion, once a medical team has been chosen, it is important to have confidence in them and in yourself. Your mantra needs to be, "I have a great plan, excellent medical team, and I am going to be one hell of a "good" patient. I will do everything asked of me and then some. I am a fighter and a survivor!"

Another ingredient to our adaptive recipe is dignity. Cancerville has a tendency to strip you of that very quickly. I strongly encourage you to hold on to that in any and every way you can. Jodi never wore the wig we bought for her. She preferred a doo rag or embracing a "bald is beautiful" mindset. And she was! She demonstrated her dignity by taking it all on the chin and never crying "uncle." Of course, there were tense and tight times—that is to be expected. But, throughout she held her head high and taught me many valuable lessons about facing Cancerville head-on.

I will encourage you to keep adjusting your attitude as you go along as we go along. When you get knocked off the horse I call Hope, dust yourself off, and get back on her as fast as you can. I know personally that it may take a while.

To sum adaptation up, you need a plan and a strategy, that slowly turns into a set of actions, that are supported by acceptance, perseverance, confidence, executed with dignity, and driven by hope, optimism, and positive attitudes. With those in your corner you will face the beast of Cancerville with beauty, which will slowly turn that beast into something more manageable, tolerable, and conquerable.

Activity 1:

List the basics of your plan below:

____

____

____

____

____

____

____

Take calculated risks. That is quite different from being rash.

—George S. Patton Jr.

By perseverance the snail reached the ark.

—Charles Spurgeon

Think about one stride at a time, and before you know it, you have gotten a mile under your belt.

—Jane Loeb Rubin

Life is not easy for any of us. But what of that? We must have perseverance and, above all, confidence in ourselves….and that this thing, at whatever cost, must be attained.

—Marie Curie

Put yourself in competition with yourself each day. Each morning look back upon your work of yesterday and then try to beat it.

—Charles Sheldon

Some people feel better when they can say, this is my situation, these are the healthcare team members I've picked, and this is what we've decided to do.

—Mary Jane Massie, M.D.

Activity 2:

How would you rate the level of confidence you have in your plan?

1   2   3   4   5   6   7   8   9   10
not confident   very confident

How would you rate the level of confidence you have in your medical team?

1   2   3   4   5   6   7   8   9   10
not confident   very confident
If this is # 5 or less you need to talk to them about it or find a new team.

Activity 3:

How would you rate the level of confidence you have in yourself?

1   2   3   4   5   6   7   8   9   10
not confident   very confident

If this # is 5 or less seek out support to strengthen your confidence.

Activity 4:

Think of other challenging times that you have faced in your life. What strengths did you draw from to adapt and rise to them?

____
____
____
____
____
____

Activity 5:

List some things you can say to yourself to keep your perseverance strong:
I will get through this and survive.
I'm tougher than I look.
I'll do what I have to do.

_______________________   _______________________
_______________________   _______________________
_______________________   _______________________

PART III

Helpful Tools from which to Draw Strength

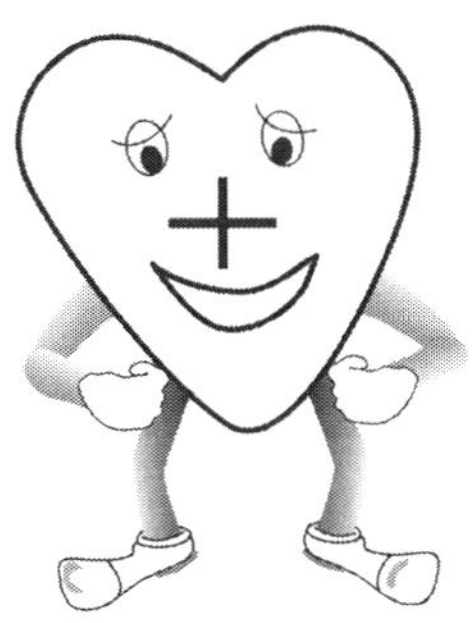

CHAPTER 8

Affirmation

Nothing fuels motivation like a positive and hopeful attitude, and nothing fuels that like affirmations. That is why in both books I wrote, each chapter begins with an affirmation. These are simple, affirmative statements such as:

- I will learn how to cope better in Cancerville.
- I am an adaptive person and have a track record to prove that.
- I aim to be "DAM STRONG!" at all times.
- I will do my best to make healthy choices on my behalf.

The words we use to speak to ourselves are very important in forming our thoughts, which lead directly to our feelings as well as our optimism. For example, if you say to yourself "Shoot, cancer! I'm finished. What a crying shame. I am terrified," it will lead you down a negative trail, make your Cancerville journey all the more difficult, and might even become a self-fulfilling prophecy. We will examine this more in the next chapter. For so many reasons, it is so much better for you to talk to yourself positively, encouragingly, and hopefully. Even something as simple as: "I will do the best I can."

Years ago I coached my son's baseball team for one season. We were "The Bad News Bears" personified. My key offensive strategy was to get them to walk around the bases. Only one boy could hit, and he showed up only occasionally. But I pumped these boys full of hope. I told them we could win a trophy if we tried really hard and believed in ourselves. I added that we needed to root for each other, play like a team, and always try our individual best.

With those words, a little luck, and more walks than one would expect in baseball we made it to the playoffs. The other team, far superior to ours, was stymied when we tied it up at one game apiece. That they won the best two out of three did not matter a hoot. We showed them what attitude could do to their competence. We made them work for their win and coming in second was not exactly chopped liver for my bears.

I have been driven many times to my knees by the overwhelming conviction that I had nowhere else to go.

—Abraham Lincoln

Regardless of how you feel inside, always try to look like a winner. Even if you're behind, a sustained look of control and confidence can give you a mental edge that results in victory.

—Arthur Ashe

Your future depends on many things—but mostly on you.

—Unknown

Many people, who don't see themselves as particularly strong or positive are amazed at how well they handled Cancerville. Unlike Lincoln, they never fell to their knees. They have said to me, "Though I was and am plenty scared about this, I actually handled it better than I thought. Sure I cried and worried, and had negative thoughts as I went through treatment, but I did far better than I would have thought, all things considered."

Clearly, you have a choice between saying "I'm a dead duck," or "I am going to be a survivor, get through this bumpy road, and live a long life." Obviously, I want you to choose the latter course. Even if the affirmations you repeat over and over to yourself don't feel believable, keep repeating them and eventually they will become part of your being. The old expression is "Fake it till you make it," and I fully and firmly endorse that prescription.

Activity 1:

I have noticed that different people can relate to different mantras or affirmations. From the list below check those that resonate for you. Try using one a day like a "vitamind!"

I will be okay.
I like me.
I will have a peaceful day today.
I will get through this.
I am a survivor.
I believe in me.
I have a great family and friend support team.
My medical team is top notch.
I am at one of the best cancer centers in the world.
I have taken charge and feel in control.
I have done my homework.
I will bounce back emotionally.
I will continue to strive for optimism and hope.
I will heal and be healthy again.
I will communicate kindly and sensitively.
My survival is my goal.
I am a good person and deserve good things to happen.
I love me.
I will take better care of me from now on.
I will be able to get through this.
My mind remains open to all possibilities.

Activity 2.

Write at least five affirmations of your own that feel right for you.

____

____

____

____

____

____

____

Activity 3:

I hereby commit to using affirmations each day as a way of creating hope, optimism, and positivity for myself despite having cancer.

____

signed

____

date

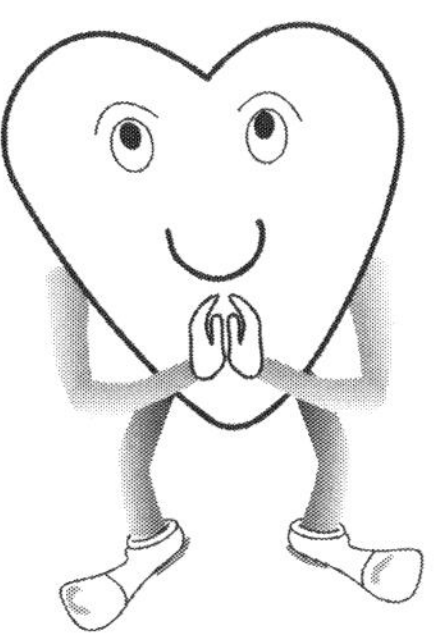

CHAPTER 9

Inspiration

That which inspires one person, conspires to annoy another. Inspiration is individualized and tailored to our nature and needs. My question to you is what and who have inspired you over the years?

For me, many have contributed to my beliefs in inspiring ways by their words and their actions—John F. Kennedy, Martin Luther King, Jr., and John Lennon to name a few. All three were imperfect in some ways, but held some ideals and ideas that were quite admirable. It is truly sad that these three inspiring men were all assassinated—mindboggling really!

Helen Keller's story inspired me as a boy, as did Abraham Lincoln, George Washington, FDR, and Harry Truman. Renowned authors such as Merle Miller, John Updike, John Steinbeck, Phillip Roth, Bernie Siegel, M.D., Theodore Isaac Rubin, M.D., and many others inspired me to try my hand at writing—and I am still trying!

Key is who has inspired you and whether their actions, attitudes, and words can help you through your Cancerville journey? I encourage you to seek them out, while also looking for new sources of inspiration. What I've discovered, in both my professional and personal life experience is that words are very powerful messengers bringing strength, courage, determination, and hopefulness right into our minds. These, in turn, translate into empowerments that fuel our being able to rise to the challenges, time and time again. Repeat after me "I'm Still Standing!"

Do you agree with Frank Tibolt's statement? I don't think I agree with the last sentence, but you decide for yourself. I was inspired to write a book for "heart and soul givers" in 2005, and five years later I took action to do just that.

It is important to note that in addition to words, music can be a very powerful source of inspiration as well. Consider, as Activity 6 encourages, including it in your daily regimen.

> *The healthcare community has become increasingly aware of the power of music to support people undergoing cancer treatment. Research cited by the American Cancer Society indicates that music has been shown to do everything from reduce high blood pressure to provide relief for depression and anxiety.*
> *—Leanne Flask*
> *Coping With Cancer Magazine*

The difference between a successful person and others is not a lack of strength, not a lack of knowledge, but rather a lack of will.

—Vince Lombardi

Far away in the sunshine are the highest inspirations. I may not reach them, but I can look up and see the beauty, believe in them, and try to follow where they might lead.

—Louisa May Alcott

You can't wait for inspiration. You must go after it with a club.

—Jack London

The best teachers of humanity are the lives of great people.

—Unknown

We should be taught not to wait for inspiration to start anything. Action always generates inspiration. Inspiration seldom generates action.

—Frank Tibolt

Activity 1:

Jot down names and/or sources of inspiration for you in the past. These could be family, friends, teachers, authors, famous people you admire, etc.

____

____

____

____

____

Activity 2:

Formulate a plan to seek out those sources of inspiration in one way or another. Sources include your personal library, the public library, internet, Amazon, etc.

I will _______________________________

I will_______________________________

I will_______________________________

I will_______________________________

Activity 3:

Think about creating an Inspirational Notebook or including, as part of your diary(see chapter 11), important inspirational messages that resonate with you so you can draw from them often. I've tried to give you many strong words of inspiration and wisdom in this workbook. Feel free to circle the quotes you like and are helpful, and paper clip the page so you can come back to them. Or, write them in your inspirational notebook.

Activity 4:

Here are some books worth reading for their inspiring content:

No Excuses
Kyle Maynard

Life on the Line
Chef Grant Achatz and Nick Kokonas

Love, Medicine & Miracles, A Book of Miracles, Help Me to Heal, The Art of *Healing, and others by Bernie Siegel, M.D.*

The Last Lecture
Randy Pausch

It's Not About The Bike
Lance Armstrong

iCanSir
George P. Kansas

No Matter What!
Jay Platt

My (So-Called) Normal Life
Erin Zammett

Tuesday's with Morrie
Mitch Albom

The Alchemist
Paulo Coelho

If Life Were Easy, It Wouldn't Be Hard: And Other Reassuring Truths
Sherri L. Dew

For those spiritually inclined here are some books that can be helpful:

The Purpose Driven Life
Pastor Rick Warren

When Bad Things Happen to Good People
Rabbi Harold Kushner

The Book of Mormon
Joseph Smith Jr.

The Power of Positive Thinking
Norman Vincent Peale

Activity 5:

Here are some of my favorite words of inspiration:

There are no coincidences in life—just endless opportunities and possibilities.
—William Penzer, Ph.D.

Nurture great thoughts, for you will never go higher than your thoughts.
—Benjamin Disraeli

It doesn't matter how slowly you go so long as you do not stop.
—Confucius

Great works are performed, not by strength, but by perseverance.
—Samuel Johnson
Gratitude is the memory of the heart.
—Unknown

Obstacles don't have to stop you. If you run into a wall, don't turn around and give up. Figure out how to climb it, go through it, or work around it.
—Michael Jordan

Breathe in the future. Breathe out the past.
—Unknown

You, yourself, as much as anybody in the entire universe, deserve your love and affection.
—Buddha

It's not what they take away from you that counts: it's what you do with what you have left.
—Hubert Humphrey

Whatever you want to do, do it now. There are only so many tomorrows.
—Michael Landon

One of the secrets of life is to make stepping-stones out of stumbling blocks.
—Unknown

The only thing we have to fear is fear itself.
—FDR

Have great hopes and dare to go all out for them. Have great dreams and dare to live them. Have tremendous expectations and believe in them.
—Norman Vincent Peale

Remember, danger is very real but fear is a choice.
—Line from the movie After Earth

Activity 6

Music, for many people, can be inspiring. I listen to relaxing music all day at my home, office, and when walking in the park. I find Barbara Streisand's albums, especially, "Higher Ground" very powerful and uplifting.

I find, however, that one person's music is another's torture. There was a dude in the park at the basketball courts today rapping away wearing an "Attitude is Everything!" tee. Not my kind of music, but my kind of guy.

Below, please identify the kind of music that inspires you and pledge to listen to some every day. Many people going through radiation or chemo, find listening to music before, during, and after—if possible—a helpful and healing relief.

My kind of music is __________________________________

____

____

My promise to myself is to listen to it whenever I can.

____

Signed

Date_____________

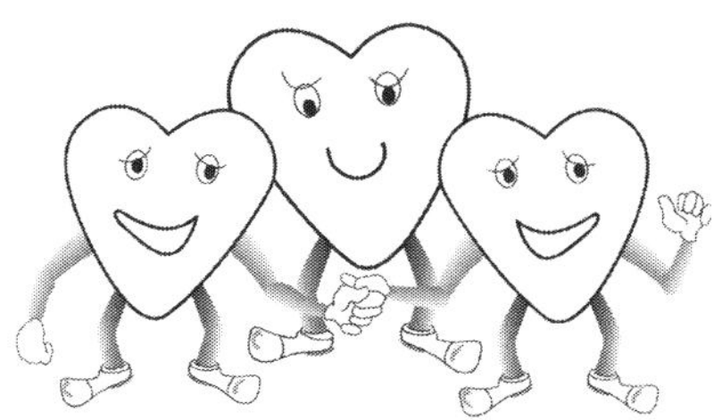

CHAPTER 10

Affiliation

Most people, in or out of Cancerville, need people. Very few can go through the challenges of life flying solo. While some need to surround themselves with people, many are comfortable and content to have a few good people on their team. A few, like myself, are pretty self-contained beyond enjoying family support. The latter is not necessarily a positive trait, as it limits one's opportunity to receive support during difficult times.

> *I vividly remember giving the eulogy for a young staff member who died of AIDs. I walked right out of the Church, past his family and my colleagues and headed back to my office a few blocks away. I sat silently for the better part of an hour, crying, reminiscing, and beginning the grieving process.*
> *When my colleagues returned several said, "You should have stayed. We all talked outside the church giving each other support, remembering Nick, and we began to heal."*
> *I always regretted not hanging around and being part of that "support group."*
> *William Penzer, Ph.D.*

I am hopeful that you are a "people person" and have a solid support net of warm and caring family and friends—the people I call "heart and soul givers" in Cancerville. If you do not, I am encouraging you to reach out in every way possible to find support and companionship on your journey. Even if you have family and friend support it won't hurt to add to your team, as the more the more helpful.

> *Cindy was a fiercely independent woman. However, when first diagnosed with breast cancer as a single mom of two young children, she needed help in a variety of ways. She called in all her "markers."*
> *Cindy said, "I asked friends and neighbors to help me get my kids to their activities when I was too sick to drive. These wonderful people— angels— made sure we had food to eat and were totally devoted. Even the kid's teachers pitched in. It was not how I wanted it to be as I*

Make new friends but keep the old. One is silver and the other gold.

—*Sung as a round at P.S. 64 in the Bronx, New York. Perhaps the only thing I remember from elementary school.*

Loneliness and the feeling of being uncared for and unwanted are the greatest poverty.

—*Mother Teresa*

A hug is a great gift—one size fits all, and it's easy to exchange.

—*Unknown*

Failure to create and maintain quality personal relationships with other humans is as dangerous to our physical health as smoking.

—*Psychiatrist Stanford University*

wanted my kids to know their mom was okay, but sometimes you just have to do what works—especially when cancer gets in your way!"

One of the ways for you to get support is to ask for it. Though this is not always comfortable, I encourage you to do whatever you need to get the help you need. Though we tend, as people, to want to be self-sufficient, cancer interferes with that in many ways. Part of your acceptance involves coping with your limitations and accepting help.

The Anonymous programs draw from the support of sponsors for those struggling with addiction A sponsor is an elder who has been clean and sober for many years. The same idea can be applied to Cancerville. Finding someone who has been through the very same type of cancer you have and is a survivor can be very helpful in many ways. They can answer questions, offer reassurances, provide helpful feedback, empathize with the difficult speed bumps, and generally guide and support your journey. Many cancer organizations maintain lists of "sponsors" willing to help the newcomer, in person, via phone, skype, etc. If that idea resonates with you seek out your sponsor and engage.

My friend Kathleen was a businesswoman when diagnosed with lymphoma. After a long and challenging course of treatment, during which she received no emotional support except from family and friends (as no professional help was available in her small community), she decided to something about it. She returned to school, received a Masters in psychology, and has worked fulltime in oncology overseeing the program and doing counseling ever since.

Last year she was diagnosed with breast cancer. Here's what she said in the Stowe VT Weekend of Hope newsletter welcome: " This year I was diagnosed with cancer again after 16 years cancer free. This was devastating and frightening. However, this time was different. I understood the benefits of support and how to ask for it….. I learned much of that by…never losing sight of the fact that having cancer can be very lonely and I don't have to do this alone."

Sometimes, the support you need is basic and practical (i.e., rides to treatment, help when showering, help with the chores and/or children, finances, etc.). At other times the support you need is more emotional (i.e., a shoulder to cry on, a pair of ears to complain to, a voice of reassurance in the Cancerville wilderness, etc.). Here are some good words when it is for the latter:

- I need to hear your voice.
- I need you to be here for me, if not physically, emotionally.
- I need someone to help me laugh.
- I need a little piece of you right now. Please call me.
- I need your help to get me though this.
- I need a friend.

From Caring4Cancer magazine comes these important words:

It is normal to feel hesitant about asking your family and friends to pitch in with cleaning, cooking, or childcare. Take comfort that these people want to help by doing something meaningful for you. Ask a family member or friend to coordinate this effort and relieve you of this responsibility.

Know that many survivors are more than willing to pitch in and lend a hand to pay it backward, forward, and sideways for the help they received and for having survived the journey—even if they don't know you. Many websites, blogs, and radio programs by survivors are helpful supports as well. Many are listed under Resources at the beginning of this Workbook.

Though it is not always comfortable to ask for help and support, just as it wasn't for Cindy or Kathleen, in certain situations (Cancerville being one of them) it is important, if not imperative, that you do. Hopefully, most of the time you won't have to ask, but I have met people who had limited people support to draw from. Not everyone has a loving, supportive partner and others who are able to care and to give. Anyone with half-a-heart will likely be responsive to a cancer patient in need. That said, there are some people who have less than half-a-heart. I sincerely hope you don't know them!

Of course, another area of affiliation and help are support groups that meet to talk or to have some fun such as bowling, yoga, etc. Included in this group are those random people you might meet in waiting rooms and treatment centers. No one understands what you are dealing with better than those people dealing with the same thing. In Cancerville, we are all friends united by the common bond of coping with the demands of Cancerville and seeking survival. The onus is on you to reach out (even if that is not your style) seeking and offering support to others. The bonds one forms with another survivor can be powerful and can last a lifetime.

Life isn't about surviving the storm; but how you dance in the rain.

—Unknown

Giving people a little more than they expect is a good way to get back a lot more than you'd expect.

—Robert Half

Trouble is part of your life. If you don't share it, you don't give the person who loves you a chance to love you enough.

—Dinah Shore

Friends are relatives you make for yourself.

—Eustache Deschamps

I still believe that love is all you need. I don't know a better message than that.

—Paul McCartney

It matters not who you love, why you love, when you love, or how you love, it matters only that you love.

—John Lennon

Activity 1:

Describe what support, practical and emotional, you would like to receive? Be as specific as possible.

____
____
____
____
____
____

Activity 2:

Who on your team of family, friends and neighbors can you truly count on?

________________________________   ________________________________
________________________________   ________________________________
________________________________   ________________________________

Activity 3:

I hope you run out of space for Activity 2. But if not, where else might you seek support and help? Circle all that apply and are comfortable:

Support Groups
Survivor Organizations
Non-profits such as American Cancer Society, Gilda's Club, Stupid Cancer, and so many more.
A mental health professional
Internet
Your medical team
Friends of friends
Church or Synagogue
Cancer Treatment Centers
Other: feel free to email me at bill@cancerville.com____________________
Other: post your needs on cancerville.com Facebook page____________________
Other:____________________________________
Other:____________________________________

Activity 4:

Embrace this mantra: "I will reach out for support when I need it!"

Activity 5:

I have many Cancerville email friends who have reached out to me based upon reading my books or hearing me speak. It is an honor to offer them some gentle support from time-to-time. Feel free to send me an email if I can be of help:bill@cancerville.com

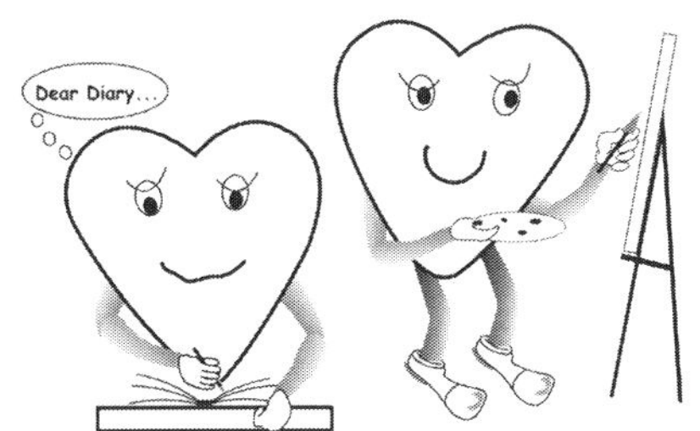

CHAPTER 11

Ventilation

Journaling

When Jodi was diagnosed in 2005 I began to journal every night. I found it to be an ideal way for me to vent the emotional cess that accumulated on a daily basis. Because I did not share my writings with anyone, I could say anything I wanted in any way I needed—and I did! Very often it was my anguished and angry scream in the night. My language wasn't always the King's English, but hey, I was venting loud and clear. That is the beauty of keeping a private journal, and why I am encouraging you to try it out.

When I wasn't venting, I became my own cheerleader. Phrases like: "chemo concludes," "hair grows back," and about being "realistically optimistic," were born there and repetitiously written in my journal. In fact, the book for "heart and soul givers" was first outlined as part of my scribbles. My writings helped me to see the value of action, distraction, and relaxation. I encouraged myself along those lines before encouraging others. In my diary of ten-plus yellow pads, I found my "voice of reassurance" that helped me to become "DAM STRONG!"

My professional experience has taught me that journaling is not for everyone, but can be very useful for many. Some people, like myself, write regularly, while others pick up the journal when the mood and need strikes them. Others just don't find it a helpful support and vent.

Jim Higley, a prostrate cancer survivor, tells an interesting story in his article published in Coping with Cancer Magazine. A friend of a friend, who was a cancer survivor, called him shortly after his diagnosis.

You may not even realize it at the time Jim," she said, " but if your mind and heart are open, I promise you will come out of this with a gift that will change your life. Your gift will be yours and yours alone. And you will never be the same. Regardless of what happens with your cancer.

I once had a writer friend who said, 'When it hurts, write harder.' Those words remain on a Post-It above my computer.

—Diana Raab
   Survivor

It is often wonderful how putting down on paper a clear statement of the case helps one to see, not perhaps the way out, but the way in.

—A.C. Benson

I write in my diary to bring order to the chaos in my life.

—Virginia Woolf

Every problem has a gift for you in its hands.

—Richard Bach

I do not like to record my dull, heavy moments in my Journal. I would like for it to record nothing but brightness and sunshine, but life is made up of light and shadows, and mine is no exception.

—*Anne Frank*

Writing was as important to my recovery as any chemotherapy or radiation I received.

—*Loree Luther*

For me, my diary is my life, my comfort, my second existence.

—*Ramon Gil Navarro*

Karen also gave Jim a notebook. "Write Jim," she said. "Take time to write." Jim says, "For the first time in days, I was excited. Karen framed my life in a way no one else could."

My encouragement echoes Karen's. Use the following pages to write and when you run out of space make copies, buy a diary, or a pack of yellow pads. Intriguingly, had Karen given me her advice about a gift, I might have not initially understood what she meant. I would have thought, "This is no gift, this is a nightmare!" Sometimes gifts take quite a while to evolve.

Actor and screenwriter Evan Handler, doesn't share the view that cancer is a gift. He says, " I was certainly opportunistic about latching on to benefits and advantages, but I would never personally say that I think my life has been better for it. I think it is fine to say I have a great life even though I'd rather all these things hadn't happened to me."

But the "gift" aka an "opportunity" that I received from being forced to deal with Cancerville-by-proxy, was the insight and understanding that led to my books. I view them as a gift to others, who unfortunately are forced to visit Cancerville too. In giving back to them, the books are a gift to me as well.

More than two decades ago, James Pennebaker, Ph.D., a social psychology researcher, discovered a very positive association between expressive writing, trauma, and health improvements.

Dr. Pennebaker states in CURE:

Our basic findings have been replicated in the last 25 years in more than 300 related studies from labs around the world. We're still not entirely sure why it works, but the result crosses boundaries of age, gender and social class .... When something unexpected or jolting occurs, such as the diagnosis of cancer, our brains automatically try to figure it out. Writing may make that figuring out process more efficient. If we can construct a story out of it, a simple and coherent story, it may allow us to move through the experience more efficiently.

An interesting footnote to my pages of journaling occurred one year after Jodi's surgery. Going forward, I wanted to try to transform July 8th—the date of her mastectomy—from a sad/bad/mad day to a neutral one of no significance. I sent Jodi, Zev, and Ronnie out with some "mad money" (pun intended), while I sat on their lovely roof garden in Manhattan, and read every word of my journals. I anticipated that my words would make me cry, but I found them interesting, but no longer emotional. My focus was on Jodi's survivorship and has been ever since.

From that day forward we have never acknowledged July 8th again—except perhaps in the quiet privacy of our minds. It is not an "anniversary" worth recalling. Most intriguingly, upon returning home I put those yellow pads in a "safe place" so no one could find them, and have no clue where they are—and I haven't bothered to look for them. My journals served their ventilating purpose at the time, and are now no longer relevant. On the following pages see if writing is right for you.

> In commenting about President Barack Obama as Time magazine's Person of the Year, Michael Sherer said, "He began to navigate the issues in the days after the election by scribbling his hopes on a yellow legal pad. Obama has always thought best by writing, and for that reason he struggled to keep a diary during his first term, a task at which he hopes to redouble his efforts over the coming years." The President says, 'In my life, writing has been an important exercise to clarify what I believe in, what I see, what I care about, what my deepest values are. The process of converting a jumble of thoughts into coherent sentences makes you ask tougher questions.'

> Then one day an idea came to me. I love entertainment, and like most people I use music, TV, and movies as a way to escape from the stressors of life. Plus, I love to write. Marrying two of my passions—entertainment and writing—was something I had never thought to do, but it seemed like a perfect combination…Let yourself be open to new things. Try things that you have never thought of doing before. Enjoy them. And enjoy yourself.
> —Francine Brokaw
> Breast Cancer Survivor
> Author, Beyond the Red Carpet

Activity 1: Use the following areas to start your journal, or get a notebook, or a whole bunch of yellow pads.

Date   Time   Title (all optional)

____

____

____

____

____

My journal is my constant companion. It is never far from my reach… It is a front porch of solace and retreat when I am tired and weary.

—Nicole Johnson

The nicest part is being able to write down all my thoughts and feelings; otherwise I might suffocate.

—Anne Frank

Open up that journal and get poetic finally.

—Jason Mraz

I am humbled that many have an interest and draw strength from my ongoing journey.

—Robin Roberts
Upon announcing her forthcoming book about her pre-cancerous blood disorder-MDS.

Date   Time   Title (all optional)

____

____

____

____

____

Date   Time   Title (all optional)

____

____

____

____

____

Date   Time   Title (all optional)

____

____

____

____

____

Date   Time   Title (all optional)

____

____

____

____

____

Date   Time   Title (all optional)

____

____

____

____

____

Date   Time   Title (all optional)

____

____

____

____

Creative Expression

Writing in a diary is only one way to vent. There are obviously many others from which to choose. Getting our feelings out, especially when they are toxic, tainted, and coated with the angst that fills cesspools, is very, very important. Holding them in causes a form of emotional constipation that actually weakens our ability to cope in strong and healthy ways. In whatever way works for you, please vent on a regular basis.

> *Jake, when he was able, made beautiful get-well cards for the other children at Memorial Sloan-Kettering. His drawings inspired the other children, and their bright colors cheered everyone up—including Jake.*
>
> *His mom, Cristina, decorated his hospital room to the nines and changed them frequently, especially for holidays like July 4, Thanksgiving, and Christmas. Her creative efforts kept everyone's spirits just a little bit brighter—especially Jake's and his twin brother and best friend, Chase. It also helped her to feel she was doing something helpful at a time when so much was "out of control" for her family and her, as she was on call 24/7 at MSK. Jake and Cristina were there for many months.*

Activity 1:

The following is a list of ways people creatively express themselves other than journaling. Please circle those that have been helpful for you in the past. Put a star next to those you have circled that you would like to try as a way of venting your feelings and expressing them creatively.

- painting
- poetry
- short story writing
- photography/videography
- sculpting
- writing essays and articles
- blogging
- tweeting
- facebook updates
- knitting, crocheting, embroidering
- stained glass
- gardening
- other_______________________________
- other_______________________________
- other_______________________________

Drawing replaced my tears, and colors gave me back a sense of belonging. While I was drawing, fear and sadness would disappear, as if I was leaving it on the paper.

—Marisol Del Sol-Auten
  Lymphoma Survivor

It's normal to feel overwhelmed by the stress of cancer when you have to adapt to so much so quickly. Creativity offers a unique tool for creating meaning and making sense of your experience.

—Caroline Peterson

Activity 2:

Go back to the above list. Put a check mark next to any activities you never tried but would like to experiment with and experience.

Activity 3:

Observe and inquire as to what family and friends do to vent their angst and see if any appeal to you. List them below putting an X through any that are of no interest.

____

____

____

____

____

____

____

Activity 4:

If you are not up to any of these activities right now, please come back to this section at a better time for you.

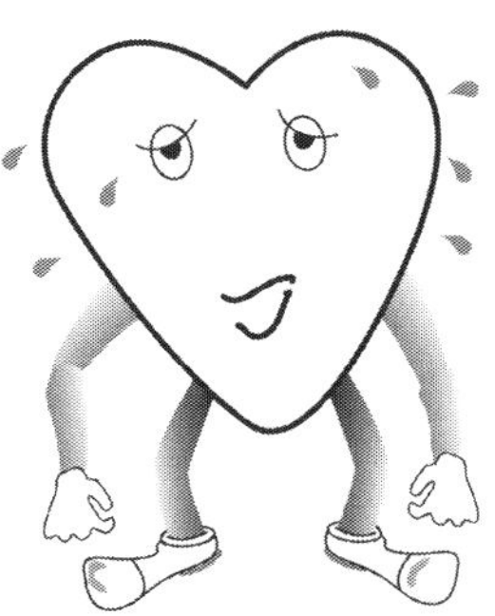

CHAPTER 12

Perspiration

Since physical activity is often a vent, I gave thought to including this in the previous section. I then decided that exercise can fit into many sections including motivation, distraction, complementation, etc. I concluded it deserved a place of its own.

Let me be clear that there will likely be times during your cancer treatments when physical activities and exercise will be last on your list of priorities. Much simpler behaviors will take center stage. I get it— I really do.

There will, however, be times when you are feeling stronger, healthier, and more comfortable. During these times, exercise that creates some sweat can be very helpful. Please check with your doctors before doing anything strenuous.

Stuart Scott, a well-known sports commentator, has battled back from stomach cancer at least twice. A few days after chemo he does his martial arts exercises to potentiate the chemo. To him, this activity symbolizes his fighting back and taking charge of his cancer, and more importantly his health. I'm quite sure, this won't work for everyone, but it does for him.

The advantages of physical exercise are well known, despite the fact that most of us are couch potatoes. But cancer is a wake-up call for many who quickly come to realize that taking better care of themselves can make a very significant difference. The "good juices" of brain chemistry and body harmony are naturally produced through exercise. The "runner's high" applies to just about every activity that produces sweat and an increased heart rate.

According to Caring4 Cancer magazine the type of physical activity you do depends upon you, your stage and type of cancer, your fitness level, how you feel during treatment, and your doctor's advice…. Listen to your body and your doctor, and do what feels right for you.

All truly great thoughts are conceived while walking.

—*Nietzsche*

An early-morning walk is a blessing for the whole day.

—*Thoreau*

If you're seeking creative ideas, go out and walk. Angels whisper to people when they go for a walk.

—*Raymond Inman*

Nobody is worth more than your body.

—*Melody Carstairs*

In addition to and perhaps because of those neurochemical changes associated with the exercise high, physical activity pumps up people's emotional chemistry. I have always said, "I don't enjoy exercising at the gym, but I do enjoy leaving the gym! I feel really good as I enter the parking lot." Exercise also helps you feel you are taking charge of your body, and doing your best to nudge yourself towards health, wellness, and survival. Though it is by no means a guarantee, people who participate in a regular exercise program tend to live longer and enjoy a smoother ride.

> *That said, I just walked two miles in the park on a beautiful sunny day in South Florida. I try my best to practice what I preach. Walking also helps me clear my head creatively. Today I realized there needed to be a chapter on communication. That is where and when Chapter 17 was born. Perhaps angels do talk to walkers!*

> *My mom went to the gym regularly until she was ninety-eight-and-a-half. She also swam regularly well into her 80's. Our whole family has a vision of her walking around our swimming pool again and again when she visited. I'm sure she would attribute her longevity (in a family not known for that), in part, to her commitment to exercise. WNP*

I'm sure my Mom and Sylvia would have been best of friends. Sylvia, a colon cancer survivor for more than twenty-five years, exercises for three hours every morning including a Zumba class. She is eighty-nine years young. Sylvia says:

> *The essence of getting better is determination….It's all about PMA— positive mental attitude. I chose not to be self-indulgent or feel sorry for myself. I made the decision to be strong, positive, and take care of myself in every possible way. That was a long time ago, and I am still going strong!"*

For a variety of positive reasons, I encourage you to be active, once you are able. Obviously, if you are already an avid exercise participant I am preaching to the choir. If physical exercise, activity, and sweat have never been your thing, consider trying it in different forms until you find something that gels with you and your comfort zone. For me, walking in the park is the best, especially if Ronnie joins me.

Movement is medicine for creating change in a person's physical, emotional, and mental state.

—Carol Welch

There's nothing sweeter than sweat.

—Linda Levritt

Happiness doesn't come from doing what we like to do but liking what we have to do.

—Wilfred Peterson

It is exercise alone that supports the spirits and keeps the mind in vigor.

—Cicero

Please remember that we are not talking marathons or triathlon's here.

Most people are not programmed like George or Stuart Scott, the "karate kid" previously mentioned. I am only encouraging twenty to forty-five minutes of doctor-approved activity three times a week in any of the following areas:

- Bicycling
- Jogging
- Walking
- Swimming
- Yoga
- Weight Lifting
- Exercise Machines
- Rowing
- Tennis/Racquetball/Squash
- Gyrotonics
- Zumba
- Pilates

While you are at it enjoy (with your Doctor's approval) a steam, sauna, or hot tub. Sweating, in any form, releases all kinds of physical and emotional toxins. However, if your immune system has been weakened, obviously avoid these till it is back to itself.

> *The American Cancer Society has published the following exercise recommendations for cancer survivors:*
>
> - *Avoid inactivity and return to normal daily activities as soon as possible.*
> - *Aim to do 150 minutes of moderate intensity or 75 minutes of vigorous intensity aerobic activity each week.*
> - *Include strength-training activities at least two days per week.*

If you are an "exercise virgin" consider hiring a personal trainer—especially one who specializes in cancer survivorship—to get you started, teach you safe and effective techniques, and help you to show up. Woody Allen said, "Eighty percent of success is showing up." When it comes to physical exercise and being active it may just be one hundred percent! You might also want to check to see if the hospital or cancer center in which you are receiving treatment have exercise programs that can guide you through the Cancerville physical activity maze.

> *Research has shown that walking for three and a half hours per week may reduce the risks of cancer recurrence and improve response to therapy. Walking may also reduce fatigue, depression, and anxiety, while improving your functional status and your quality of life.*
>
> *—Julie Dial*
> *Coping With Cancer Magazine*

> *Sandra Wade describes that she endured a marathon of chemo and radiation for inflammatory breast cancer. By the time treatment was completed she was almost an invalid at age fifty-two. After researching her options to build up her strength, she learned that Jupiter Medical Center in Florida (not far from our beach apartment) offered help by therapists trained in cancer Survivorship Training and Rehab (STAR Program). She says, "I am doing everything on my own. I exercise at home now. I am dressing myself, cooking, cleaning and getting in and out of the bathtub."*

He who could learn to fly must first learn to walk and run and climb and dance; one cannot fly into flying.

—Nietzsche

Inactivity related to cancer and its treatment can contribute to systemic problems, including loss of strength and muscle torque as well as negative effects on the respiratory and cardiovascular systems.

—CURE

Winning isn't everything; it's the only thing.

—Vince Lombardi

Activity 1:

In the space below, write you plan to engage in physical activity once you are able.

MY PLAN FOR EXERCISING AND GETTING MORE FIT IS TO:

____
____
____
____

Activity 2:

Here is what I have been able to do since I have been given the green light by my body and my docs to exercise. If now is not the green light, come back to this one—hopefully soon:

DATE____
DATE____
DATE____
DATE____
DATE____

Activity 3:

Here is my pledge and plan to continue and commit to maintaining an active exercise regimen, within my physical capabilities and limitations:

____
____
____

Signed_______________________________________

Dated____________________

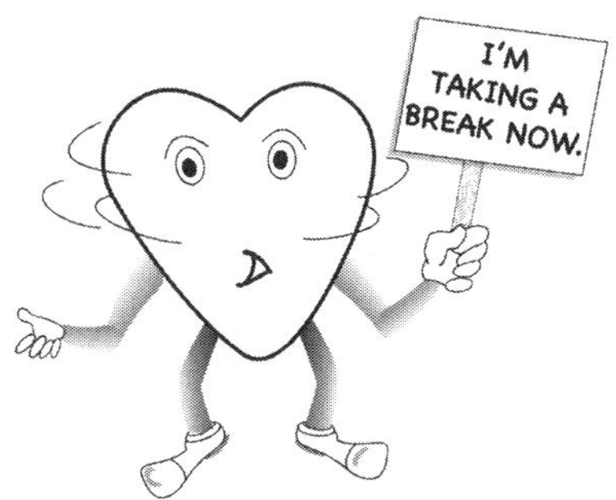

CHAPTER 13

Distraction

There will be times, perhaps many times, when you will need to take a break from Cancerville. There are a Heinz variety of ways to distract yourself, and there is no way I can cover them all here. Mostly, the distractions you gravitate toward will be those that feel right for you. I am not big on movies or TV so it is unlikely that I would seek those out, if I was ill and needed to distract myself from time to time. My wife Ronnie is the opposite.

Then again, one never knows. I might decide in that moment of discomfort and distress, to see all of the important movies I missed along the way. Or, I might choose to finally view the "I Love Lucy" dvd reruns we bought several years ago, watched three, and then abandoned the rest to a drawer. Since laughing in any health zone is helpful, Lucy's silliness would be a welcome relief.

Some distractions are internally generated and some externally. Right now, as I type, I am distracting myself through internally generated activities. If I were to turn on the TV and watch a football game, my distraction would be external. My guess is that some of us are internal distracters, some external, and some combinations of both. An important question, which I will soon ask is what is your type?

By using your preferred distracters, you can build temporary windows and exit doors through which you can breathe fresh "emotional air" and experience a brief respite from the riggers of Cancerville.

Several years ago, I was feeling rather robotic because I was working all the time. Out of a sense of frustration I asked myself a simple question: "What did I like to do when I was a frivolous kid and not focused on accomplishment?" The answer popped out of my mind immediately. "Play basketball."

Holding aside my lack of talent, I bought one and began shooting solo at the park in which I walk. I have continued to do that and enjoy that very much. My shots, unguarded as they might be, are far better than as a teen.

The point is that it is not about the ball. It is about us all finding enjoyable distractions to spice up our lives, and get us through the rough patches we inevitably encounter, especially while making our way through Cancerville.

Activity 1:

Circle which of the following are things you have enjoyed doing in the past and might find helpful now:

TV
Movies
CDs/DVDs
Email
Facebook
Twitter
Google/ Web Searches
Reading
Listening to Music
Playing Music
Art Projects
Puzzles/Crossword/Seduko, etc.
Shopping
Writing
Knitting/Crochet/Embroidery
Photography
Board Games/Online Games
Exercise in any form
Golf
Cards
Bingo
Other:_______________________________
Other:_______________________________
Other:_______________________________

Activity 2:

Of those you circled, place a check next to those activities that are realistic for you to do now.

Activity 3:

Of those you circled and checked, put a star next to at least 3 activities that you are doing or would like to commit to doing for purposes of distraction—more if you like.

Activity 4:

Use this space to come back to and update any new distractions you try or discover. Note whether they were discovered by you or by some external influence.

____
____
____
____

Activity 5:

Note any distractions that were generated by others (i.e., lunch/movie invites, visits/gifts, etc.

____

____

____

____

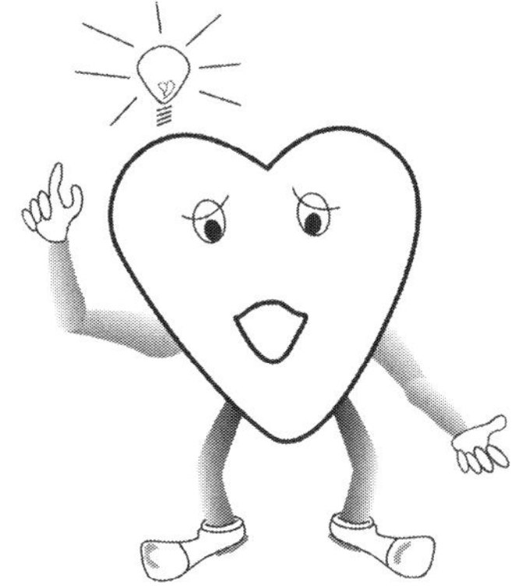

CHAPTER 14

Imagination

One of the many reasons our minds are a "slingshot" is that they are filled with a vast array of useful materials, tools, and potential resources. One of these is our imagination—our mind's ability to create. Though some people may be more creative than others (i.e., Michelangelo, Shakespeare, Mozart, Franklin, Edison, Freud, Spielberg, Jobs, and the woman who wrote the Harry Potter series to name just a very few) you possess creative juices of all kinds as well. The purpose of this section is to encourage you to use them fully to counterbalance the demands of Cancerville.

Let's understand that our imaginations can work against us as well. People can be quick to imagine negative events and catastrophic consequences, especially under challenging circumstances like cancer.

Upon being diagnosed and throughout his treatment, Tony was convinced his life, as he knew it, was and would continue to be totally different. His imagination took him to dark and scary spaces as his "creativity" was all negative and foreboding. Even thoughts about re-experiencing past pleasures were creatively twisted into sad anticipations in the future. It took me a while to help him move to "assuming" he would be okay, especially since he had been given strong reassurances by his doctors. Many people, like Tony go for worst-case scenarios at a time when they need to hold onto best-case ones.

Another example of unhelpful imagination is people who decide they will be okay without traditional treatments. That creative interpretation, in most cases, is "fools gold" that typically turns out to be dangerous. Obviously, you are free to make your own choices based upon your beliefs. However, I have met or heard about too many people who choose to do nothing, or do only risky and under-researched alternative treatments who did not survive. Then again, I have met a few people who swore by their alternative regimens that they felt saved their life. I simply urge you to be a cautious consumer in this confusing zone.

I would much rather you use your imagination to picture positive outcomes and relaxing experiences. Or you can use your imagination to take yourself out of Cancerville from time to time and "escape" to neutral or more comfortable zones.

Commitment unlocks the doors of imagination, allows vision and gives us the 'right stuff' to turn our dreams into reality.

—James Womack

I am certain of nothing but the holiness of the heart's affections and the truth of the imagination.

—John Keats

Reality leaves a lot to the imagination.

—John Lennon

Dreams are today's answers to tomorrow's questions.

—Edgar Cayce

There are no rules of architecture for a castle in the clouds.

—G.K. Chesterton

A good dose of fantasy is exercise for your sensibilities; it keeps your avatar strong.

—Michelle E. Goodrich

Here are some tools for you to draw from:

Changing the Channel

One of the tools I offered Tony was to use his invisible remote to switch the channel from negative programming to neutral, if not positive thoughts and images. It is not always easy to find your remote, (don't even bother to look under the couch pillows), but once you do it can quickly take you out of dark spaces to put your imagination to work in a more positive and creative fashion. Or, you can watch replays of past happier scenes and allow them to provide you with healing energies.

Guided Imagery

When feeling relaxed, close your eyes and take yourself to a calm space. It might be one to which you have been previously (i.e., grandmas house, the beach, Disney World, a cruise, the mountains, etc.). Or, take yourself via your imagination to someplace you have never been to but associate with peace, calm, and comfortability (i.e., a lake house in New England in summer, a boat ride on the Seine in Paris, a fishing trip for salmon in Alaska, etc.).

Picture yourself, in your mind's eye, being there. Take in the sights, sounds, and sensations (i.e., feel the sand beneath your feet, smell grandma's perfume, see the water off the back of the ship, or the snow on the mountains. Or, imagine how it feels to have a large fish on the line, a warm sun shining on the lake or river, snorkeling in Bora Bora and seeing the beautiful, colorful fish, etc.

There are many CDs to help you do this including mine Tranquility: *Zen and Now*, or DVDs including mine on Iquassu Falls in South America—a most tranquil space. I will send one or both upon request at bill@cancerville.com for the cost of shipping.

Fantasies Are Free

Want to be President of the United States or a major company? Want to be a rock or movie star, or a Pulitzer prize winning author? Want to be a model or builder of award winning airplane models? How about being a porn star, successful politician, or have your own TV talk show? Rather be a NASCAR driver or librarian? Through your imagination, you can enjoy being whomever and whatever you want—at least in your mind.

At appropriate times, I encourage you to let your mind and imagination run free and even wild toward whatever fantasies will help you feel happier and more comfortable. Pick a quiet time, perhaps just before falling asleep or upon awakening. Choose a positive scene, like an author writing a novel or screenplay. Create images on your mind's TV screen and hear words that make the fantasy vivid and real. Enjoy the feelings that go along with these happy, exciting, and prideful mind "movies." When you are ready come back to reality, knowing that what you created was a fictional, but no less pleasant experience that distracted you from the heavies of Cancerville.

Know, as well, that you can return to this fantasy anytime you like and/or create others that can be equally pleasing and relieving.

Important to note is that fantasies are free as long as we don't act on them. Imagining winning millions of dollars in the Powerball lottery and figuring out how you would spend those gains is pure fun. Going out and buying more tickets than you can afford based upon that fantasy is far from free. Take note of all those important people who took their fantasies into their real lives, and were tarnished as a result, not to mention costly legal fees, loss of position, image and prestige. To draw the full benefits of fantasies, they must remain as such.

Imagine a Brighter, Warmer, Prettier Space

Not all Cancerville facilities are pleasant looking. Some are in serious need of an upgrade and makeover. In fact, some of the most prestigious cancer centers in the world get A+ for caring expertise and D- for facilities. In situations where you can't spruce up the place a bit like Cristina did for Jake's room, you can use the power of your imagination to make it look better.

See beautiful pictures of pleasant and colorful scenes where drab walls are bare. See a window looking out on a lovely garden filled with brightly colored flowers on a windowless wall. See a cascading waterfall in the waiting or treatment room, and hear the sound of the water as it flows down and hits the base. Use your imagination in creative ways to "remodel" the spaces you visit in Cancerville if need be.

You may think I am encouraging you to have visual and auditory hallucinations. That is precisely what I am doing! However, I am doing that in your best interest so you can see and hear pretty images and sounds where none exist. Just as you may bring a device (i.e., smart phone, ipod/pad, laptop, etc.) to see and hear comforting images and sounds during treatment, so can you do the same in your mind, drawing from your imagination whenever you want. Remember always that your mind is a slingshot and needs to be used as such at critical times.

Laugh A Little

Though having cancer is no laughing matter, laughing matters a great deal in Cancerville and in any challenging situation. There is much data, both anecdotal and experimental, to show that laughter can release healthy brain chemicals, facilitate healing, reduce pain, vent pent-up emotions, and ease tension levels.

Clearly, the joke needs to be appropriate and sensitive to the serious circumstances. Just as a well-placed line in the middle of a sermon or even eulogy can break the tension, so can a chuckle in Cancerville. Sometimes it is a joke shared with others, and other times it is a personal laugh or giggle.

Imagination is as good as many voyages—and much cheaper.

—George Curtis

Imagination lit every lamp in this country, produced every article we use, made every discovery, performed every act of kindness and progress, created more and better things for more people. It is the priceless ingredient for a better day.

—Henry Taylor

Imagination will often carry us to worlds that never were. But without it, we go nowhere.

—Carl Sagan

Imagination offers people consolation for what they cannot be, and humor for what they actually are.

—Albert Camus

If you can't make it better, you can laugh at it.

—Erma Bombeck

No one is laughable who laughs at himself.

—Seneca

If we all did the things we were capable of doing, we would literally astound ourselves.

—Thomas Edison

Normality is a fine ideal for those who have no imagination.

—Carl Jung

The best way to predict the future is to invent it.

—Alan Kay

Rob literally laughed out loud as he rode alone in the elevator at Memorial Sloan Kettering Hospital. It was a Saturday morning and he was very eager to see his young son Jake, who was hospitalized for treatment to overcome the most serious form of childhood leukemia. I am pleased to repeat that Jake overcame all of the odds and is doing fine today.

What caused Rob's laughter was that he realized he had inadvertently entered the elevator reserved for religious Jews on the Sabbath— it automatically stopped on every floor. Rather than cursing or bemoaning his slowed down fate, this Catholic man just chuckled until he finally arrived at Jake's floor, and could greet his son with a big smile on his face. The joke was on Rob and he loved it!

In Cancer Today magazine, Brenda Elsahler tells of the time she was in the hospital when a nurse came in with a hypodermic needle. The nurse made her laugh and she didn't feel the needle at all. Throughout her Cancerville journey she says laughing helped her with both her physical and psychological pain. Her article says, "We've all heard that laughter is the best medicine, and research has now backed it up scientifically.

Imagine Distancing Yourself from Cancerville

Okay, I won't lie to you. Unfortunately, you will never leave Cancerville behind and be rid of it completely. You can, however, put much distance between yourself and your cancer experience.

If you are currently going through treatment, try to picture in your imagination, a time when your treatment is completed and you are a "survivor" in the complete sense of that term. This is not a fantasy, but a reality in the making. I don't like the "new normal" idea for many reasons, but I do like the idea of continuing your life without the demanding intrusions that Cancerville can impose. Though you may have to make some adjustments and adaptations, hopefully, you can reclaim your life as it once was.

See a time when cancer is just a footnote to your life, rather than your main focus. See that you are done with doctors and treatments, but for an occasional check-up. See yourself finally feeling better and resuming your day-to-day life, enjoying yourself, being able to be fully productive again, and having learned a variety of life lessons that you can apply for many years to come. Please keep picturing these images while combining them with your voice of reassurance, even though you may be in active Cancerville mode for a while.

Activity 1:

Briefly list times in your life when using your imagination was helpful and pleasant for you:

____

____

____

____

____

Activity 2:

Of the imaginative activities suggested above, please list them in order of your ability to relate to them.

____

____

____

____

____

____

____

Activity 3:

Identify some scenes for guided imagery experiences to which you can best relate. Feel free to draw from scenes not given as examples as well.

____

____

____

____

____

Activity 4:

If being creative and imaginative has never come easy for you, try any of the following to stimulate your drawing from these tools:

Pay more attention to creativity in your everyday life (i.e., signs, TV advertisements, emails, or Facebook posts).

Take a risk and experiment privately with any of these ideas, or others that feel more comfortable.

Use your imagination for brief periods of time—as short as 20 or 30 seconds to start with.

Find images in magazines or on line that resonate with you, and use them to drift off into mental imagery, fantasy, etc.

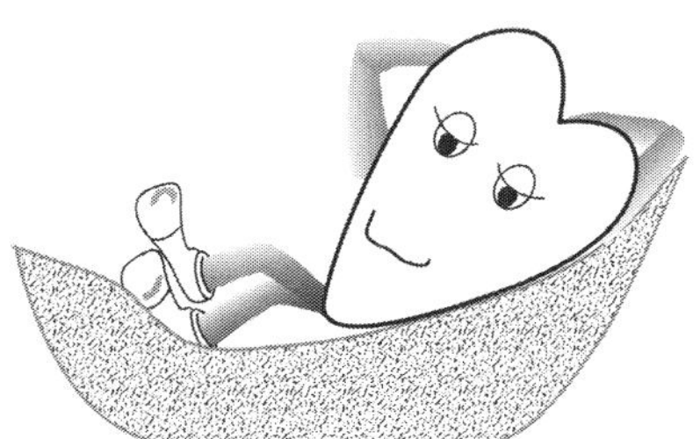

CHAPTER 15

Relaxation

What would Freud say about my saving this chapter to be written last? Probably, that my wires are twisted, and what most people find relaxing, I find tedious and vice versa. In my somewhat warped mind, work has always been more like play, and play more like work. Such is the nature of relaxation, so that one person's Omm is another's OMG. Undeniably, how you relax is your choice, as long as it isn't dangerous to your health, hurtful to others, or against the law. I can hear someone saying, "Gee Bill, your no fun at all." Guilty as charged! Feel sorry for Ronnie!

Here I want to "sell" you on using specific relaxation tools and techniques throughout your Cancerville journey and beyond. Before treatment, during treatment, and after treatment, relaxation tools soften the impact. As you already know, there are many choices from which to pick. There are CDs, DVDs and apps— many for free. There are healing words and music that you can download onto your phone, laptop, or Pad. They help with mental and bodily distress, pain, and so much more. They distract from the scene at hand, enable sleep, and help you to wake up in a better mood, with increased energy, even on a "not so good" day. They can also prepare you for the demanding treatments, so you can approach them in a calmer, cooler, more comfortable fashion.

My encouragement is simple. Check out the sources and forces of relaxation. Look around at what is available and go for it—at least to try and experiment. Somewhere out there in the universe, there is a tool or a few for you, that will feel right and facilitate a more comfortable state of body and mind. Achieving that will make your Cancerville journey just a little easier to bear.

I repeat that there are many CDs to help you do this including mine Tranquility: *Zen and Now*, or DVDs including mine showing relaxing video of Iquassu Falls in South America—a most tranquil space. I will send one or both upon request at bill@cancerville.com for the cost of shipping.

Activity 1:

Here are some other sources of relaxation tools:

soundings.com
drmiller.com
newagemusicgarden.com
live365.com
weber.com
soundsleeping.com
innerhealthstudio.com
everydayhealth.com
relaxationdirect.com
naturalhealingtools.com

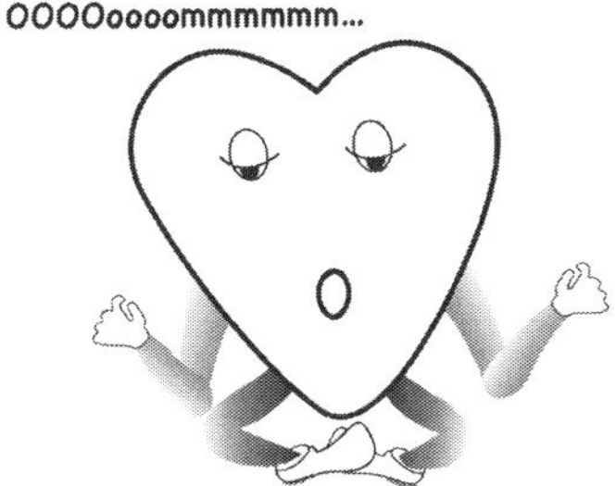

CHAPTER 16

Complementation

On January 1, 2013 I wrote on my mindlymatters.com blog, "There is nothing more important or of greater priority on your 'to do' list than taking better care of you." This applies especially to people dealing with cancer.

Having cancer is a wake-up call, not only about your death potentials, but also about your life potentials. The question we can all ask ourselves is, "Am I taking care of me to the best of my ability?" If the answer is "NO," now more than ever you need to evaluate how you can be taking better care of you, while you deal with all the stresses of your life in Cancerville.

So-called complementary treatments can help you to do just that.

Realistically, they are not so much treatments in the medical sense, as they are treats in the mind/body sense. Here is a partial list of activities that, with your doctor's approval, can help you to heal:

- Yoga
- Mindfulness
- Meditation
- Self-hypnosis
- Acupuncture
- Massage
- Progressive relaxation
- Guided imagery
- Support groups
- Healthy nutrition
- Reiki
- Exercise
- Spirituality
- Journaling
- Creative activities
- Cooking
- Gardening
- Hot tub/ sauna/steam
- Travel
- Movies/TV
- Music
- Fountains
- Candles
- Other *Visiting spiritual and peaceful places*
- Other____________________________
- Other____________________________
- Other____________________________

Information abounds in books and online about these calming activities. Finding tranquility in Cancerville is not always easy, but all of the above offer that very possibility—at least from time to time.

In my travels around the world, I have observed that entering a holy or peaceful place offers an automatic, invisible force that relaxes me. It could be a temple in Kyoto, Japan, a mosque in Istanbul, Turkey, a synagogue in Venice, Italy or a gothic church in Paris, France. Or, it could be the Morakami Gardens in Delray Beach, Fl, The Botanical Gardens in the Bronx, New York, or enjoying a picnic at the beach, countryside, or along a river bank. My simple point is that placing yourself in peaceful space from time to time is a refreshing counterbalance to the intensity and tensions of Cancerville.

Please note that in this chapter and throughout the book I stayed away from even mentioning nutritional issues, special diets, and supplements because they are complicated and controversial. Follow your doctor's guidance and advice in all areas, along with your own "gut" feelings. Check out the second edition of the American Cancer Societies' *Complete Guide to Nutrition for Cancer Survivors.*

An analysis of 18,000 participants has shown that acupuncture is effective for treating chronic pain in four specific areas.
—Cure

Yoga has earned accolades as a complementary therapy and now studies are confirming its value.
—Claudia M. Caruana

Mindfulness practices can help cancer patients to settle their minds and get grounded in present-moment experiences and give them a sense of control when it seems like many other aspects of their lives are beyond their control.
—Susan Bauer-Wu, Ph.D.

Activity 1:

Put a check next to any in the list on the previous page that you are currently doing. Add it to your pride bank.

Activity 2:

Circle any activity in the list not checked that you would like to try soon.

Activity 3:

Please commit to the following statement:

I _______________________________________promise and pledge to take better care of me in every way I can from this point forward—forever.

____
signed

____
date

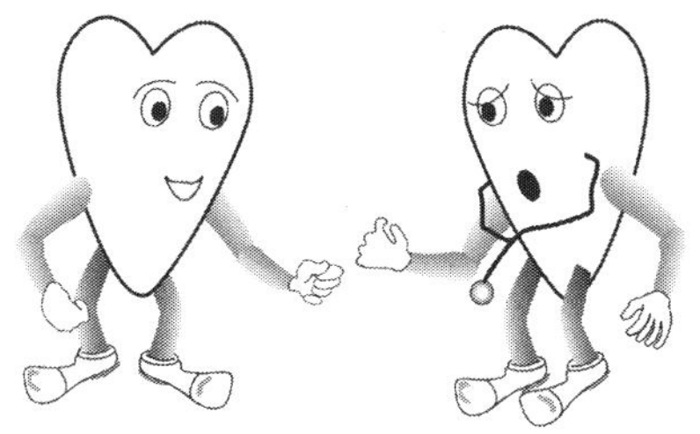

CHAPTER 17

Communication

There are so many different forms of communication in Cancerville that it makes it difficult to generalize. All media, social and otherwise, are likely to be used by you throughout your journey. Communication will range from interactions with strangers or friends of friends, to your closest family and friends, to a variety of medical professionals—more than you ever wanted to meet!

You will be communicating about things you never dreamed you would, while wishing for the mundane and routine conversations of old. Let's hope and assume you will be back to them soon. In addition, you needn't be on "cancer call" 24/7. You are allowed and need to talk about other things.

> *You have the right as a patient to expect your doctor to be competent, to be assured that he or she is knowledgeable and technically skilled. However, you also have the right to expect caring and compassion from your doctor…. Three C's form the cornerstone of good doctoring: competence, compassion, and caring.*
>
> —*Jimmie C. Holland, M.D. and Sheldon Lewis*
>   *The Human Side of Cancer*

It is critically important that you be able to have positive and productive communication with your medical team. They are your ombudsmen and women—your important guides on your Cancerville journey. They are also your most important source of information as they are the experts. Forge a solid communication with your caregiver team and they will help you on your journey.

> *When actress Maura Tierney was asked, "What helped you cope with your breast cancer experience?" she replied "Arming yourself with information is really helpful. I trusted my doctors, and I spoke to them a lot. If anything was bothering me, I would call and ask them."*
> *Coping with Cancer Magazine*

Constant kindness can accomplish much. As the sun makes ice melt, kindness causes misunderstandings, mistrust and hostility to evaporate.

—*Albert Schweitzer*

Silence is deadly. We have to talk about it.

—*Charlie Wilson*
  Prostate Cancer Survivor
  Singer/Songwriter

Feelings are everywhere—be gentle.

—Eric Hoffer

Your family and friends should understand that you need space. Just be honest and tell them in a nice way that you need some time to yourself.

—Gwendolyn Otey

The reason dogs have so many friends is because they wag their tails and not their tongues.

—Unknown

Man does not live by words alone, despite the fact that sometimes he has to eat them.

—Adlai Stevenson

Much has been written about the silly/inappropriate things people can say to you when informed of your diagnosis. For most people, serious illness, disability, and the like are awkward topics that arouse their anxiety, which leads to those less than fine and fitting comments. I will help you practice stock answers that get your message across without unleashing your rage. Almost always, I believe such people don't mean to offend or upend. If, however, one of your team members is toxic, then you will need to have a serious chat, distance yourself, or disconnect. But, start by giving them the benefit of the doubt.

If you have a toxic member of your team, have them read " help me live: 20 things people with cancer want you to know" by Lori Hope (great name and good book). Herself a lung cancer survivor for several years, she was direct and forthright in admonishing people in the "heart and soul giver" position on what to say and what not to say.

Here is a taste: "I want compassion, not pity." "Advice may not be what I need, and it can hurt more than help." "I love being held in your thoughts or prayers." "I need you to offer support to my caregiver, because that helps me too." " I am still me, treat me kindly, not differently."

I think you need to establish clear boundaries, while not making communication so tangled and confusing as to leave people puzzled as to how and what to say. Strike a reasonable balance in all zones.

There is no denying that communication in Cancerville can easily go south. This is true of any life zone that is filled with stress, pressure, ambiguity, and tension. Cancerville is all of that and more, so there will be times when interactions go right off the track. You need to be prepared for that and have some ways to quickly repair the miscue or misunderstanding.

From How to Cope Better When You Have Cancer:
… communication in any emotionally charged area, especially in Cancerville, can quickly deteriorate in destructive ways. With stress and cess flowing forcefully in Cancerville, communication can easily come undone. Under these pressures and upsets, communication with medical personnel, family, friends, work associates, and even strangers can quickly go off-track like a model train going at too high a speed. Fighting in one war zone is more than enough for you to handle. Let's work together to prevent creating any other combative areas.
—William Penzer, Ph.D.

Here are some common causes that trip the switches of conflict, confusion, or miscommunication:

- Adults communicating like a critical parent to a "bad" child.
- People yelling/cursing/calling names to another.
- Putting someone down in other ways.
- Taking a black and white view on a subject that doesn't fit that perspective.
- Displacing anger and angst onto innocent people trying to be helpful.
- Inappropriate comments at just the wrong time, and sometimes, appropriate comments, also at just the wrong time.
- Misunderstandings of the "I thought you meant…" kind.

> *Marty Clarke, P.A.-C, Ph.D. gives his cancer patients the following five rules for dealing with family and friends:*
>
> 1) ***Don't tell me to have a positive attitude.*** *Just because I don't feel good, cry, express unhappiness, anger, or confusion about having cancer doesn't mean I have an attitude problem.*
> 2) ***Don't tell me to eat.*** *If I don't eat enough, it's only because I can't. I understand that I need food to recover. I promise to eat as much as I can.*
> 3) ***Please don't ask me how I feel or how I am doing.*** *All day long I work very hard at forgetting how I feel and how I am doing. I just want to enjoy being with you and doing the things I can.*
> 4) ***Don't give me your advice.*** *Everyone gives me advice. I find this overwhelming and disturbing. I don't know what to do with all of this advice, much of which is contradictory. So, if I want your advice I will ask for it.*
> 5) ***I have the right to remind you of these rules.***

Craig T. Pynn, a prostate cancer survivor, talks about jumpers (focus on happy endings) minimizers (focus on high cure rates) and fixers (focus on prescribing what he should do.) All of them annoyed him, and seemed to simplistically leave out the complex decisions he had to make, procedures he had to endure, and unknowns with which he had to wrestle. He says:

> *By focusing on the caring intentions that lay behind their words, I could see they meant only the best for me. As time went on and they recovered from the initial shock, most of the jumpers, minimizers, and fixers eventually became sympathetic—even empathetic—listeners. Had I made the sarcastic responses that so greatly tempted me when I heard their comments, I would have hurt both them and me. In this instance, I was glad that I had chosen to be patient.*
> *—Caring for Cancer*

He who cannot forgive others destroys the bridge over which he himself must pass.

—George Herbert

The first to apologize is the bravest. The first to forgive is the strongest. The first to forget is the happiest.

—Unknown

The genius of communication is the ability to be both totally honest and totally kind at the same time.

—John Powell

Clearly, Ms. Hope and Dr. Clarke are giving you, the patient, permission to establish clear boundaries to protect you from the annoying and irritating communication, well intended as they may be, from those around you. I encourage you in the same direction, using your most assertive, adult, and peace-making voice when needed. Mr. Pynn demonstrates the value of patience, and doing your best to avoid confrontation and hurt feelings.

The more you are able to draw from your strong, adult-based voice, the more those around you will stay in theirs. The problem is that when you are tired, weak, and feeling like crapola, (my editor was shocked to learn that this is a real word) staying in your adult voice is easier said than done. I encourage you to try your best to do that whenever you can. My hope is that the people around you—caregivers and "heart and soul givers"—are sensitive and responsive to your needs, so that communication can stay on-track.

Activity 1:

Repeat after me:

"I have the right to not be upset by well-meaning people who say annoying things, and will calmly offer feedback to make sure that doesn't continue to happen."

"I will do my best to stay in my calm, rationale, adult voice, but I reserve the right to 'lose it' at times, just because I need to."

"If there is a person who refuses to follow my lead and continues to be toxic, I will distance or disconnect myself from them, simply because I just don't need any added stress at this time."

Activity 2:

What will you say if someone gives you advice that you don't want or need?

____
____

What will you say if someone asks how you are feeling?____________
____

What will you say if someone tells you a cancer horror story?_________
____

What are some stock statements you can have available when someone annoys, upsets, or irritates you in other ways?____

____

____

____

____

Activity 3:

What are some ways you can express appreciation for support, help, and constructive caring, and empathic communications?

____

____

____

____

Activity 4:

Write down some good words to stop digging the communication hole deeper, once things have become conflicted and are headed in the wrong direction?

Let's take a time out.
I don't have the strength to fight with you.
I need to go lay down for a while.

other____

other____

other____

other____

PART IV

Helpful Encouragements from which to Draw Strength

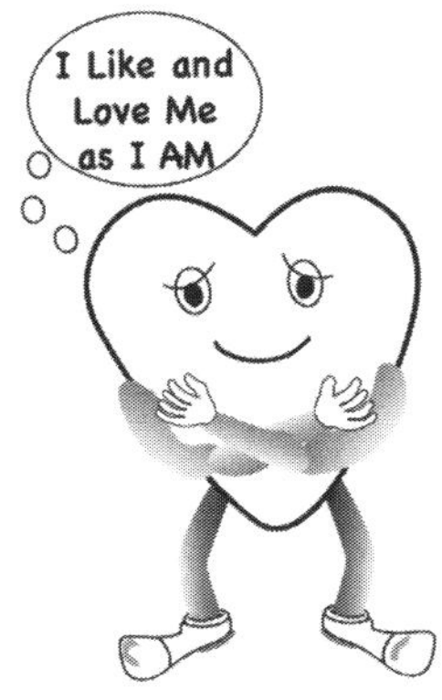

CHAPTER 18

Self-Imagization

I wish I could give you an infusion, if not a transfusion, of self-esteem to fill your self-image and self-confidence full. I wish it was that easy to fill in the holes in your self that have been left by journeying through Cancerville. Unfortunately, it is not. Given your unique history, nature, and cancer experience, recreating a healthy sense of self will likely be a unique challenge—but definitely a doable one.

There is much talk about rebuilding self-image and self-esteem in articles and books, a few seemingly superficial suggestions, and not much else. While hanging with friends, taking a yoga class, or enjoying a bubble bath can be pleasant and healing, they can sometimes add to one's self-consciousness and dis-ease, which can diminish a survivor's self-esteem. These typical suggestions to enhance self-esteem also reflect simplemindedness about a complicated topic. My goal is to clarify self-image issues, as well as to guide your journey toward reclaiming your positive sense of self. Even if you are feeling good with you this chapter is worth your read.

> Once treatment ends, you may feel pressure from others to move on and to not worry about changes in your appearance. However, it takes time to adjust to and accept your post-cancer body, and it's important to do so at your own pace. Acknowledging your feelings about your body and how it works for you can help you maintain a positive self-image during and after treatment.
> —Carrie Panzer, LCSW

> *The real voyage of discovery consists not in seeking new landscapes, but in having new eyes.*
> —*Marcel Proust*

What Are We Talking About?

What exactly are self-image and self-esteem? Though these words are used frequently, they are typically not clearly defined. Here is my effort to give you a sense of what these words mean. Your self-image is the sum of how you see yourself as a person in terms of every important life area. It is defined by how you see your physical, emotional, intellectual, financial, relationship, and health state. This subjective self-assessment takes into account your accomplishments relative to your goals. It is as if you have an inner pair of

Make a pact with yourself today to not be defined by your past. Sometimes the greatest thing to come from your hard work isn't what you get for it, but what you become for it.

—Steve Maraboli

Beauty comes in all sizes—not just size 5.

—Roseanne Barr

Pain is a pesky part of being human…. I have also learned that because of pain, I can feel the beauty, tenderness, and freedom of healing.

—C. Joybell

eyes that view and judge you. Though you may not share those views with others, you are acutely aware of the plusses and minuses that they represent.

The subjective sum of that evaluation translates into your self-esteem. Your self-image and self-esteem combine to form the basis of your self-confidence, which is a very important component of your success in all life zones. Unfortunately, for many people, their self-image is undeservedly low (i.e., I'm too short, tall, fat, thin, dumb, poor, etc., etc., etc.).

Many filters can distort a person's inner gaze and cause one to feel lesser than, inadequate, self-conscious, and down on oneself. It is easy, too easy, to lose sight of the qualities that one brings to the table of one's life and diss oneself unfairly. Quite often, the roots of a poor self-image, lower than deserved self-esteem, and resulting lack of confidence go deep within the bowels of one's life. Negative programming that likely occurred in one's youth can leave an indelible but powerful residue of self-deflation. In many instances, early life and family trauma have defaced the billboard of your self-image. Those scars need to be healed too, along with your newly acquired physical and emotional cancer-related scars.

Clearly, one's self-image and self-esteem are a complex equation influenced by many subjective factors. Understandably, cancer can add a new multi-layered destructive dimension to your view of you.

The Impact of Having Cancer on Issues of Self

For obvious reasons, cancer rarely enhances one's sense of self. The physical and emotional scars left in its wake are significant and traumatizing. For most people the unknown is always daunting, but ever more so after being diagnosed and treated for cancer. Being a survivor is undeniably pride-worthy, but also a gnawing reminder of having been to a place no one really wants to have visited.

The younger you are when diagnosed, the more having cancer and the treatments you have undergone can affect your self-image and self-esteem. In most instances, cancer leaves its mark on your body and your mind, not to mention the ever-present worry that it can come back. It can also interfere with your life, causing self-consciousness and questions about careers, dating, sex, fertility, finances, etc. If some or all of these have occurred, you need a plan to wrestle back your sense of self to a more positive level.

This is not to imply that if you are older when diagnosed you emerge from the rigors of Cancerville unscathed, as that is hardly the case. Issues of body image, the impact of harsh treatments, the desire for longevity, and the uncertainty of it all affect all age groups. Even in midlife and older, having cancer interrupts and interferes with the flow of your life—and very often that flow was challenging enough before cancer.

No one easily tolerates what we psychologists call a "narcissistic injury." Not to be confused with a selfishly associated narcissism, such wounds wreck havoc with our psyches. Just recall for a moment how devastating a couple of pimples were when you were a teen. People's self-consciousness and what I call "the what other people think syndrome" do not disappear just because someone is older. Our child and teen parts of our self typically live on as long as we do.

Losing hair after treatment is difficult, even though usually hair grows back. Losing a limb or other body part is obviously traumatic because they don't grow back. Even with reconstructive surgery, it is often an imperfect imitation of the original. Ditto with prosthetic devices. Of course, for the many who struggle with body and self-image issues even before they are diagnosed with cancer, the effects of cancer and its treatment only add to that heavy burden. Believe me when I say, though I am not insensitive to your upset, you are more, much more than your body parts.

The Core Ideas that Can Help Rebuild Your Self-Image and Self-Esteem

Recognize that everything in life is relative.

While I was devastated and down during my 31-year-old daughter's chemo for breast cancer, my friend Ben called one morning. His words, "I envy you, Billy," caught me off guard. I asked, "How can you Benjy, you know what I am going through?" He replied, "Cause my daughter, who just turned 18 last week, was killed last night in a horrible car accident. She was an innocent passenger in the back seat. At least Jodi has a chance—a good chance in today's world."

Amid my grief for my friend and his family, I was reminded of what I already knew from being a psychologist for more than forty years. Every crisis is relative to every other one. As bad as things can be, there are much worse stories out there in the "jungles" of our world. The more clearly you accept this, the less likely you will fall into a self-pity-party trap. The latter can easily work against your self-renewal efforts.

Accept that bad things do happen to good people of any age.

Life can be harsh and hurtful for no reason. Accept that unfortunately and unfairly it happened to YOU. Focus on survivorship, your future, and reinventing yourself in every way you can, in an even more empowered way. Acceptance of your situation paves the way for taking meaningful actions to lift your self-image and self-esteem.

> Diana was 18 when diagnosed with sarcoma of the hand, necessitating the loss of two fingers. She lived with shame for much too long—20+ years. During all of that time she made up stories about car accidents that never happened, hid her hand, avoided dating, and ran from Cancerville by living in an exaggerated and distorted denial. After attending a workshop sponsored by Stupid Cancer for other young survivors, she realized that she was not alone, that she could show her missing fingers openly as a survivor, not a loser, and she could finally, finally accept herself as a whole person despite her Cancerville wounds.

Life isn't always amazing: there will be times of trial and times of struggle along the way…. Be strong, believe in yourself, and show life that you are going to make it no matter what it throws at you.
—Unknown

Outside show is a poor substitute for inner worth.
—Unknown

A negative thinker sees a difficulty in every opportunity. A positive thinker sees an opportunity in every difficulty.
—Unknown

Some people make victims of their disadvantages, while others are victimized by their disadvantages.
—Robert Schuller

Self-pity is an acid, which eats holes in happiness.
—Earl Nightingale

> *Things don't change, only the way you look at them.*
>
> —Carlos Castaneda

> *When you change the way you look at things, the things you look at change.*
>
> —Wayne Dyer

> *Do not let what you cannot do interfere with what you can do.*
>
> —John Wooden

> *Courage: The most important of all virtues because without courage, you can't practice any other virtue consistently.*
>
> —Maya Angelou

> *Keep your face always toward the sunshine, and shadows will fall behind you.*
>
> —Walt Whitman

The message of Diana's story is the importance of reclaiming your selfhood much more quickly than she did. The really good news is that she finally did.

Keep in mind cancer is not the only experience that deals out difficult hands that must be played strongly in the poker game of life.

My friends' daughter was born with half an arm. From very early on she had to define her SELF in a slightly different way. Despite her absent limb, she became a champion ice skater and later a coach, an artist and sculptor, a lifeguard, and a college grad and teacher. She married her college beau and they are still happily together after many years, enjoying their two beautiful and healthy daughters.

Just look around you at all the troubles in the world and you will see that people not only redefine themselves post-trauma, but can thrive as well. Kyle Maynard was born with four half-limbs. That did not stop him from becoming a high school wrestler and, if you can believe it, football star. Read his book *No Excuses* to gain inspiration.

At the end of the day, we all need to work with what we have, not what we wish we had.

Adapt to whatever changes have taken place.

By definition, human beings are amazingly adaptive creatures. We are programmed to find new ways to tackle challenges in just about every life zone. It often takes a while, but our learning curve for adaptation is quite remarkable.

Assume that you have what it takes to take on these major changes to your life. Assume that you will figure it out. Assume that you will grow rather than shrink from your experience in Cancerville. I have met many people who have not only adapted, but have gone on to rebuild their lives in even more meaningful ways.

Bruce languished in self-pity and OMG post-treatment for about six months. He worried obsessively about his future. I pointed out to him that he was so focused on the future and its unknowns that he was forgetting about living his life in the here and now. He finally got that, made a decision to buy a home in the mountains, and is committed to enjoying everyday in everyway.

Truth be known, as the newspaper reflects daily, all of our futures are uncertain. As I have previously said, "There are many paths to Heaven only one of which is cancer."

Reevaluate your goals, dreams, and aspirations.

Are your goals the same as before Cancerville or have some shifted? Have you moved on from the proverbial Ferrari fantasy to simply want health, peace of mind, financial stability, pride bank deposits, and the like? Go forward with your updated charter for your SELF and those you love.

I have had the privilege of meeting many survivors who eventually found ways to give back to others dealing with cancer.

> As previously mentioned, my friend Kathleen was a successful businesswoman when she went through a difficult treatment for lymphoma. She needed professional emotional support, but none was available in her small town in Vermont. Post-treatment she returned to school, obtained a Masters in Psychology, and now works full-time at a hospital coordinating their oncology support program and helping patients deal with cancer. She is so pleased and proud to do for others what no one was there to do for her.

I have also had the privilege of meeting many survivors who realigned their goals and dreams in ways that had nothing to do with cancer.

Learn from your Cancerville journey.

There are many life lessons to be learned from having any serious disease or dealing with a major crisis. So often, it puts into perspective what we can so easily forget.

As one example of an important lesson, it is much more difficult to sweat the little things—the proverbial "small stuff"—after dealing with cancer.

> While our daughter was going through chemo and we were in NYC to keep her company, Hurricane Wilma hit our neighborhood hard. Phone reports of the damage to our yard and home sounded grim. We could not fly back for several days as the South Florida airports were all closed. How upset or concerned were we? Not at all! Compared to the demands and damage of Cancerville, the damage to our home was unimportant. It was just "stuff" that could be repaired or replaced.

Work toward redefining you in terms of self-image and self-esteem.

Allow your attitudes to slowly shift to encompass a broader sense of self that defines your worth as more, much more, than deformity or disease. Focus on your personal qualities that make you unique, special, accomplished, and loveable (i.e., intelligence, humor, sensitivity, strength, caring, etc.).

You never know how strong you are until being strong is the only choice you have.

—Unknown

Moving on with my life is one of the hardest things I've had to do. But in the end I know it will be one of my greatest accomplishments.

—Unknown

We learn the most important life lessons the hard way.

—Unknown

Try to transition from superficial to substantive. You probably do that much more easily for others than you do for yourself. You deserve at least the same concern, support, compassion, and understanding that you give to those around you.

> *No person is a finished thing, regardless of how frozen or paralyzed their self-image. Each one of us is in a state of perennial formation. Carried within the flow of time, you are in coming to be who you are in every emerging moment. Life is a journey that fills out your identity and yet the true nature of a journey remains largely invisible. Inside each journey a secret harvesting is at work.*
> —John O'Donohue
>   Author, Beauty

As previously mentioned, it took Diana much too long to incorporate and integrate her damaged self-image into a fairer and more positive self-esteem—but she ultimately did. Peer support helped her and can help you as well. You are not alone in Cancerville and the available resources today are most impressive.

Turn your energies toward healing your inner-self and soul.

Usually, our bodies heal slowly pretty much on their own. Our minds require some healing behaviors, which can include but go well beyond bubble baths and the like. Seeking counseling, finding a life coach, joining a support or therapy group, reading inspiring books and articles, journaling, meditating, using affirmations, and similar activities have helped many survivors recover and reclaim their self. These activities can also help update the billboard of your self, erase some of the graffiti, reduce exaggerations and distortions, and paint a much brighter and more accurate image of your current SELF.

Healing is an individualized experience, so feel free to experiment and explore what might work best for you. You are on a mission to find your SELF after a very challenging time. Please try to be patient with yourself. Healing does not come from a smart phone app or a pill. It takes some time, so take your time.

Beyond your body and your mind lies your soul. It is there that most of the transfusions of self-image and self-esteem take place. Go there often and talk softly to your soul with the same compassion and support that you would offer someone you loved in a similar state of turmoil. Healing, self-esteem, and self-loving are all very closely aligned.

John O'Donohue, a wonderfully insightful and absolutely brilliant Irish poet and philosopher, wrote some special and lovely non-religious soul-healing blessings that can help nurture and nourish you (*An Abundance of Blessings: 52 Meditations to Illuminate your Life, To Bless the Space Between Us: A Book of Blessings).*

> *In parched terrains new wells are to be discovered.*
>
> *Every life is braided with luminous moments.*
>
> *Seeing is not merely a physical act; the heart of vision is shaped by the state of soul.*
>
> *—John O'Donohue*

Let's just move forward!

A while ago I read a simple but powerful story about a South Florida teen. She was changing classes at her high school when a car ran into her. She lost a leg as a result. Here is what she said at a news conference upon being released from the hospital:

> *If I keep working at it and practice, I think I'll get through it…. The thought never really occurred to me to, like, wallow in self-pity. I just thought, it's happened. There is nothing I can do. Let's just move forward.*

It is important that you see this challenge as a necessary, doable, and transformative transition. You are special. Cancer hasn't taken that away. In fact, it has made you even more special as a survivor. Embrace that and just move forward.

Feeling empowered by your experience enables you to move forward in a stronger and more significant way than ever before. It can help you to become the most self-confident and self-loving person you have ever been, with a positive self-image and solid self-esteem. Being a survivor of anything suggests a prideworthy strength of will and determination.

See an invisible diploma being given to you on behalf of Cancerville. Let us assume and pray that you are a graduate. I believe you have learned many life lessons from having had cancer and, like so many other survivors, can apply them to the different parts of your SELF that will further enhance the rest of your life's journey.

(Portions of this chapter appeared in an article "Rebuilding Your Self-Image and Self-Esteem After Cancer Treatments." in Coping with Cancer Magazine).

Happiness is not the absence of problems; it's the ability to deal with them.

—*Steve Maraboli*

Sometimes staying strong feels impossible but giving up is not an option!!!

—*Unknown*

It ain't over till it's over!

—*Yogi Berra*

Even facing the big challenge of cancer do not give up—keep on moving, keep on living, keep on dancing.

—*Valerie Harper*
  Dancing With the Stars contestant

Activity 1:

How would you rate your self-image at this moment? (Circle one)

Very Good   Good   So-So   Poor   Very Poor

If it is less than good write down five things from the above suggestions/ideas that you can implement to feel better.

____
____
____
____
____
____

Activity 2:

Can you draw from things that you have employed in the past that helped you to feel better about yourself?

Yes______   No _____

If Yes write down some specific examples of past ideas/activities/behaviors that helped you see yourself in a better light. (i.e., went bike riding, read an inspiring book, sought counseling, talked to myself in a rational and calming voice, talked to friends, etc.).

____
____
____
____
____
____
____

Activity 3:

The above represents a billboard about your pre and post-cancer self-image issues. From the following list of positive attributes please write on the billboard the # of those qualities and characteristics that are part of your positive self-image.

1.Attractive
2.Intelligent
3.Athletic
4.Caring
5.Successful
6.Wealthy
7.Compassionate
8.A Leader
9.Life of the Party
10.Introspective
11.Social
12.A Good Friend
13.Detail Oriented
14.Creative
15.Street Smart
16.Intuitive
17.Charming
18.Good Manners
19.Achievement Oriented
20.Fun To be With
21.Strong
22.A Survivor
23.Inspiring
24.Humble
25.Other___________________________________
26.Other___________________________________
27.Other___________________________________

Now, from the following list of self-negations place a check in pencil next to any that you feel applied to you pre-cancer.

1.Fat
2.Short
3.Unattractive
4.Skinny
5.Bald
6.Dumb
7.Poor
8.A Reject
9.A Geek
10.Sloppy
11.A Loser
12.Unsuccessful

13.Not As Good As Others
14.Inadequate
15.Impatient
16.Anxious
17.Depressed
18.Lost
19.Overwhelmed
20.Other_______________________________
21.Other_______________________________
22.Other_______________________________

If those you checked still feel as if they apply add the # to your billboard in a way that shows how they deface, negate, or diminish your positive attributes (i.e., use a red pen or write the # in a way that eclipses or overlaps a positive attribute, etc.).

Activity 4:

Your goal and challenge is to work toward erasing those self-negations from your billboard if they are unwarranted or correct and eliminate them if they are true but unwanted.

Activity 5:

If you are unable to accomplish this on your own seek outside support (i.e., life-coach, counselor, group, books, cds, etc.).

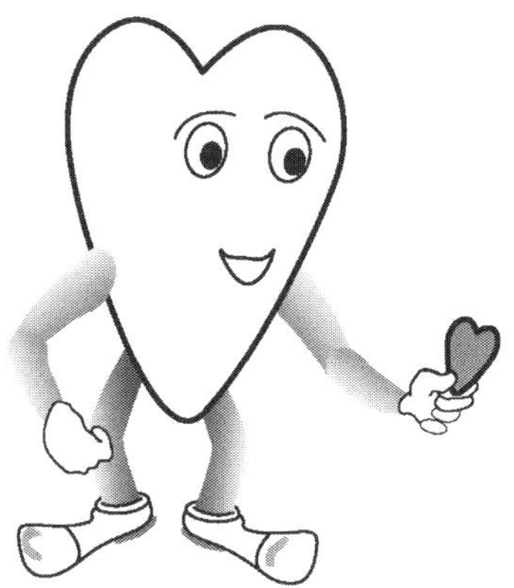

CHAPTER 19

Contribution

Many people, myself included, having been to Cancerville as a patient or "heart and soul giver," do some things to give back to it. There is something about "paying" it forward, backward, and sideways that is healing and empowering. My writing three books are all about that. At the time of the first book I said to my family, "If I help one person it will have been worth the effort." I am pleased and proud to share that I have helped many people navigate Cancerville just a little bit stronger than they might have done on their own.

> But writing is only one piece of my paying back. I plan to go to and speak at two or more conferences a year to reach out and help people in Cancerville face-to-face. But that is not all. I sponsored a team for the Relay for Life in Plantation FL—Team "Dam Strong!" In Memory of Debra Gutterman, M.D., my cousin who passed from cancer in 2010. We raised over $6754.11 for the American Cancer Society. We also see people with cancer or their family members for free or reduced fee at our Humanistic Counseling Center in Ft. Lauderdale. I am also working to raise money for Stupid Cancer to expand their support and program base. In every way I can, I will devote the rest of my career and life to helping people in Cancerville. I am a "man on a mission!" and that fills my "pride bank," while slowly emptying my "piggy bank." (lol but true!)

Apropos of the last statement, if one of your fantasies is writing a book about your experiences, I wish you luck, but would caution you to do some research first. Self-publishing has flooded the cancer book market, the costs to bring a book to life add up, and the time it takes is significant. As Ronnie said after the book for the patient came out, "Please don't write any more books." "Why not?" I asked confused, "I have so many more in my head." "We can't afford it!" was her simple response. That was before I wrote this one, so you can see how well I listen to my bride of almost fifty years. The again, as we will see, there are so many other ways to contribute to Cancerville—but if that is your dream, by all means follow it.

Compared to my relatively small contributions, so many have done so much more than I could ever do. Check out the Susan G. Komen for the Cure

---

It's not how much we give but how much love we put into giving.

—Mother Teresa

We are made kind by being kind.

—Eric Hoffer

Blessed are those who can give without remembering and receive without forgetting.

—Jeremy Fitzgerald

What is more mortifying than to feel you missed the plum for want of courage to shake the tree?

—Unknown

No one is useless in this world who lightens the burden of another.

—Charles Dickens

founder, Nancy Brinker, herself a breast cancer survivor, whose sister Susan passed from breast cancer. SGK's impact is both preventive and research-based, having raised almost two billion dollars, since they began. It is truly sad that the organization stumbled on the issue of Planned Parenthood, but that in no way diminishes Nancy's or SGK's powerful influence of raising people's awareness of breast cancer, and providing funds for research, as well as practical support all over the world.

Similarly, Debbie founded the Can't Stomach Cancer organization, which recently changed its name to Debbie's Dream Foundation: Curing Stomach Cancer (curingstomachcancer.org) Its mission is to raise money, encourage research, and provides support for people with stomach cancer. Until her personal experience and creative efforts, this was a most neglected cancer, with hardly any outreach or support.

Lance may have erred on the bike, but has raised much money and support for Cancerville through the Livestrong Foundation, so he definitely "wins a trophy" in that area in my book—literally.

In Chapter 21 I will tell you about Todd's contribution through the legacy website that he and his friend, Diptesh have built—ZarpZ.org.

Then again, there are so many individual efforts. Wendy heads the Plantation, FL Relay for Life that raises about one-hundred-and-fifty thousand-plus dollars a year for the American Cancer Society. She became involved after her sister passed from melanoma many years ago. Ironically, her husband Sam had throat cancer five years ago. To help her husband, she drew upon the very ACS resources she had helped fund all those years. Wendy and Sam are both "all in" for contributing to Cancerville in any way they can. As you will recall, "There are no coincidences…" That is why they modeled the t-shirts I created, which you can check out at cancerville.com.

There is also a cleaning woman in South Florida who cleans houses of people in Cancerville for free. Then there is Doris who came up with a "giving back" idea while sitting in her daughter's hospital room after treatment for breast cancer. Doris founded a group of older women who knit and crochet scarves, shawls, and caps to help keep hospital and hospice patients warm.

For understandable reasons, Jake and Chase's family have become ardent supporters of the Leukemia and Lymphoma Society, raising tens of thousands of dollars every year and participating in the Lite the Nite walk in Westchester, N.Y. Just recently, this family has created "Five For Fighting" with the mission of raising awareness and funds for pediatric blood cancers.

Diem Brown, a reality TV star, was diagnosed with ovarian cancer at age twenty-two, and again six years later. At her lowest point she created MedGift.com, a registry of items that people need during treatment and recovery. "I created my passion at my absolute most depressed, lowest moment. It gave me hope while I was going through treatment."

I literally just returned from the OMG Stupid Cancer Young Adult Summit (stupidcancer.org) where I met some wonderful people. The organization aims to support young adults dealing with cancer and their "heart and soul givers." It was founded by Matthew Zachary, a highly creative, energized, and driven man with a purpose—to help others who are walking in footsteps he once traveled, at a time when there were few resources of support.

> *In 1995, at age twenty-one, Matthew was diagnosed with a pediatric brain cancer and told he would not likely make it six more months— so much for medical predictions! At the time Matthew was a college senior, a music composer, and concert pianist.*
> *Side effects of his treatments limited his use of one hand. Though he still composes and plays music, he turned his creative juices into founding this amazing organization, and growing it by leaps and bounds. Still expanding its reach and outreach of loving assistance of all kinds, today it is the largest support organization in the United States for young adults with cancer. Clearly, Matthew and his mighty, albeit small band of organizers, have turned their respective lemons into a wonderful blend of lemonAID!*

The choice is clearly yours. Some people run as far away from Cancerville as they can. That is both understandable and okay. Others, however, like myself, get something back from giving back. If that works for you cool. If not, it is definitely cool as well. This is why there are no activities for this chapter. Most importantly, be well, be happy, and enjoy every day of your life, in any and every way you can.

> *Consider doing something positive with your (breast) cancer diagnosis. It takes some time to reestablish your emotional well being, but once you have found your path, helping other women with breast cancer allows your emotional wellness to soar. Some breast cancer survivors have gone on to work as volunteers in their treatment centers or local hospitals. Some have developed cancer support programs in their hospitals where none existed previously, and others have gone on to build national support programs. Find what ignites your passion, and go for it.*
> *—Dr. Linda Sutton*
> *Coping with Cancer Magazine*

In one way or another, giving back epitomizes an opportunity to heal, pay back, and contribute meaningfully and lovingly to those making the difficult and demanding journey through Cancerville.

Happiness doesn't result from what we get, but from what we give.

—*Ben Carson*

When nothing seems to help, I go and look at a stonecutter, hammering away at his rock, perhaps a hundred times without so much as a crack showing in it. Yet at the hundred-and-first blow it will split in two, and I know it was not that blow that did it, but all that had gone before.

—*Unknown*

I met Mike when he co-hosted a radio program (powerfulpatient.org) on which I was interviewed about my Cancerville efforts. Since being diagnosed with Renal Cell Carcinoma in 1997, he has become very involved with survivorship and advocacy for patients and their "heart and soul givers" in numerous ways—much too many to list. In addition to his state and national involvements with cancer organizations and survivorship issues, Mike is active in his community, conducting programs for the elderly and the terminally ill, and making presentations on cancer awareness and support to many organizations. Now that is what I call giving back!

In addition to giving back to Cancerville, some survivors find other avenues of contribution. Being a survivor can awaken our hearts to the importance of support at a difficult or trying time. My email friend from Scotland who is dealing with breast cancer there said, " Thanks again for taking the trouble to email me- little gestures mean big things at times like this."

So many survivors choose to reach out to other worthy causes to help make a difference. They might visit a nursing home, volunteer at the Humane Society, local Church or Synagogue, food bank, etc., etc. Research clearly shows the many positive benefits of helping others that include reducing depression and anxiety, feeling happy and energized, and increased "pride bank" deposits. Whenever we give to others in meaningful ways, it usually pays back meaningful dividends!

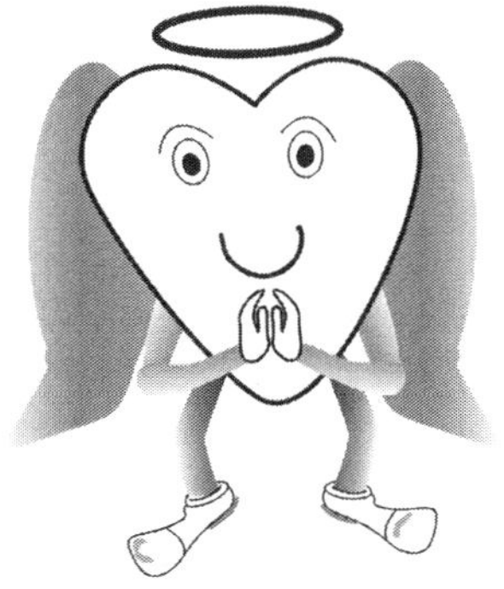

CHAPTER 20

Spiritualization

I don't know if there is really such a word as spiritualization, but it is an idea and ideal worth pursuing. It simply encourages a belief in invisible forces that influence our lives. It is accepting that miracles, blessings, and meant to be moments influenced by the angels can and do impact us. Spiritualization is about keeping an open mind to all kinds of possibilities. Bernie Siegel, M.D., is quick to say that "the more open our minds are to miracles, the more likely they will happen." Let's remember that what made Bernie's book in the '80s so groundbreaking, was that he was a scientifically trained surgeon—well ahead of his time. He taught us well.

On the train back from Bernie's house in Connecticut to my daughter's apartment in Manhattan, I had a long time to think about how those forces had already influenced my life. From the improbable meeting of my wife Ronnie on a High School trip that neither of us belonged on, to staying together through thick and thin to celebrate our fiftieth anniversary December, 2013, to our two biological sons David and Michael, and our adopted daughter Jodi from Korea, to our three wonderful grandchildren. But that only scratches the family surface.

There's the part about this nonstudent getting a Ph.D. of all things, a wonderful job as a psychologist at IBM to awaken me from my sheltered upbringing in the Bronx, the chance move to Florida, my switch into the clinical side where I have enjoyed a forty-year career of helping people through the choppy waters of life.

Then again, I was drowning in those very waters when Jodi was diagnosed in 2005, and forces greater than myself guided my path until I could get my footing on the sand, to do better coping with this complex journey. I can only wonder what forces guided my words to write the books to help people in Cancerville, including this one. Or what exactly influenced us bidding and going on that amazing trip to Africa, where Jodi and Zev were married in a Maasai Village in Tanzania.

Which takes us to one of the greatest miracles of all. Post-chemo Jodi was told that after five years of Tamoxafin she could try to conceive a child, but the odds were slim, as chemo ages reproductive organs by as much as ten years. At thirty-seven that was a long shot. Sometimes, in and out of Cancerville, the odds have nothing to do with it. Our beautiful granddaughter was born a week before Thanksgiving in 2012, and we had much to be thankful for that year and every year. With our grandsons, age

Hope is the thing with feathers that perches in the soul.

—*Emily Dickinson*

At any moment, you have a choice, that either leads you closer to your spirit or further away from it.

—*Thich Nhat Hanh*

The hardest arithmetic to master is that which enables us to count our blessings.

—*Eric Hoffer*

The only devils in this world are those running around inside our own hearts, and that is where all our battles should be fought.

—*Gandhi*

18 and age 16, our family is complete. Together they represent our miracles and blessings facilitated by the angels.

But enough about me, as this is your journey. Amid the turmoil of your cancer diagnosis, I would like you to reflect on the blessings and miracles that have happened to you. I would encourage you to feel grateful for them despite this turn in your road. Mostly, I would like you to believe that you will get through Cancerville, learn some life lessons along the way, someday put some distance between you and Cancerville, and survive the journey, even if it is against all odds.

Though I can't guarantee a miracle for you, and I would be quick to say they don't come often enough, I want to believe that yours will be coming very soon. I want you to believe that too, because as I have said repeatedly, riding through Cancerville on a horse I call Hope, can make the journey just a little bit easier to tolerate. Hope helps us to cope! It also may help us to survive. Though it is not meant for you to know your destiny, it is possible that you can use your mind to influence its direction.

Furthermore, if you are fortunate enough to be a religious person, you probably already embrace this enlightenment. Please keep in mind that even if you are not religious, you can have or develop a spiritual mindset. I surprised myself at our granddaughter's baby naming the Sunday before Easter. When Zev was talking about naming her after my mother Sadie, he said, "She was a very special person and we wish she could be here today." I automatically interrupted him and said, "She's here, she is definitely here." Thanks Bernie for your guidance, and thanks Mom for coming to the celebration!

I offer no activities for this chapter. It is a journey that you will do on your own, in your own way, and in your own time frame or not do. If you decide to take that journey, I wish you Godspeed.

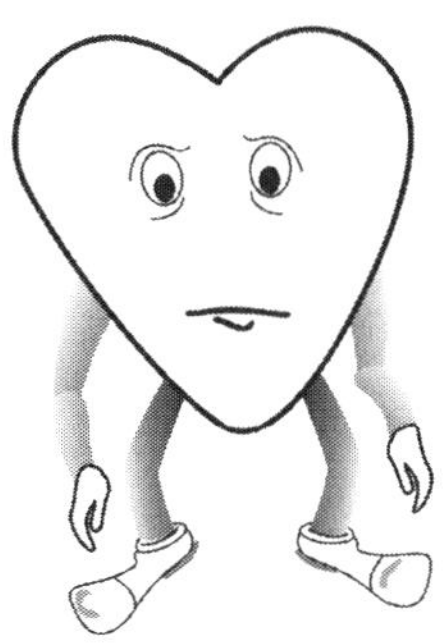

CHAPTER 21

Finalization

So, now we come to a difficult topic to even think about, let alone talk about. I have pushed hope throughout these pages like a drug dealer, and now I must shift gears. The fact remains, that for all of us, it is ultimately hopeless, as we shall all die, sooner or later. Prepare to watch me sway on the tight rope of life and death. In this regard, Cancerville sends mixed messages of survival and loss. But so does life! Cancerville is just another place filled, if not flooded, with the unknown, the unpredictable, and the doomsday. Inevitably, however, we lose our lives in a garden variety of ways.

Every day, in every imaginable, and sometimes unimaginable way, people die. They are the old and the young, the innocent and the brave, the risk takers and the fraidy cats. They die from diseases of all kinds, accidents of all types, and from guns, knives, and other weapons. As I have said, "There are many paths to Heaven only one of which is cancer."

Death has stalked my family like a serial killer. I was eighteen when my father died of a heart attack at age forty-nine; twenty-five when my father-in-law died at age fifty-one of heart disease as well. And so it went. Perhaps that is why I wrote the treatise below when I was a young man.

On Life and Death

While most of us fear death in one way or another during the course of our lives, rarely, if ever, does one hear mention of the more tragic possibility of not ever having lived. Being alive, we naturally take for granted the facts surrounding our existence and do not consider the awesome possibility of never having been conceived or born. To ponder the improbability of one's own conception after the fact is a little like betting on a horse after the race is over to be sure, but since we are not wagering but discussing, it would appear to be a meaningful endeavor.

Without going into the statistical aspects of life, consider if you will, the various physiological and situational forces relevant to your own existence. Think about the tremendous odds that existed at the time of your conception against your being conceived. Further, consider the

I don't want to achieve immortality through my work. I want to achieve immortality through not dying.

—Woody Allen

The only thing I regret about my life is the length of it. If I had to live my life again, I'd make all the same mistakes—only sooner.

—Tallulah Bankhead

Life is uncertain so eat dessert first.

—Ernestine Ulmer

Do not take life too seriously. You will never get out of it alive.

—Elbert Hubbard

You only live twice. Once when you are born and once when you look death in the face.

—Ian Fleming

I do not fear death. I had been dead for billions and billions of years before I was born and had not suffered the slightest inconvenience from it.

—Mark Twain

Death ends a life, not a relationship.

—Mitch Albom

You can't do anything about the length of your life, but you can do something about its width and depth.

—Evan Esar

overwhelming odds that existed at the time of your conception against your being conceived as you. You, if you are male, could have been born a female and vice versa, and then in all probability you would not have been you. To carry this one step further, you, as you know yourself, could have ended your semi-non-existence as menstrual blood—never to be conceived and never to be born.

Consider for a moment the fantastic luck that you had to have in order to be in a position where you could fear death. And now, once in that position, rather than fear the end result, why not applaud the beginning and silently thank whoever or whatever was responsible for giving you the privilege of dying. For inherent in this privilege is life itself and it is a privilege that many more don't have than do. To die after living is far better than to "die" without living for although in the latter, one has no awareness of death, neither does one have the awareness of life.

WNP
1964

Aren't you glad my prose has become less prosaic? Much as I encourage hope and optimism in life generally, and in Cancerville in particular, I am neither naïve nor indifferent when it comes to the very harsh reality of people dying from cancer. The numbers are hard to ignore—they scream out the facts of such losses. That is why I call my philosophy realistic optimism and recognize that miracles, blessings, and the like are not necessarily everyday events—BUT THEY DO SOMETIMES HAPPEN.

There is a built-in, natural human tendency to deny our death potentials.
Pulitzer prize-winning author, Ernest Becker describes this mechanism in depth in The Denial of Death. I found a copy of this book in my Mom's bathroom (which she called her "library") when I was cleaning up her apartment after she went into a nursing home with dementia. Obviously, at ninety-nine, mom was trying to prepare for her imminent demise.

In reality, all people, in or out of Cancerville need to do the same. But we tend not to do that. Less than a quarter of the population sign up for pre-need funeral arrangements, despite many valid reasons to do so including:

• Relieving family of that burden
• Protecting family at a vulnerable time from being taken advantage of

- Discounted fees
- Having some say over your trip to Heaven
- A reduction of anxiety by taking control of the end of your life

Mom did seek a pre-need funeral plan and had definite ideas about what she wanted, including paying for it herself despite my offering to do that. But, since she came from a family not known for longevity, that she waited to sign-up until age ninety-five to do that reflects her own denial.

Because of the traumatic impact of so many early deaths in my family, I dictated my own eulogy into a tape recorder on my thirty-fifth birthday. I wanted to "take charge" and even my otherwise silent psychoanalyst said, "Who better than you?" I am pleased to report that tape has long been gone and so far I am not yet gone. I have dictated my last wishes for my family to follow, which includes a Cristal Champagne party. I might as well go out in style, and if there is any way to do it, I will have a few sips on my journey.

The sooner we accept that we will die, the sooner we can make peace with that finality and plan accordingly. It also can help us live in and enjoy the moments and each additional day we are given. Undeniably, having a serious disease like cancer raises your consciousness, but does not have to lead to your hopelessness or despair. There are so many inspiring stories in Cancerville that give us reason to not give up. Here are a few:

> *David's kidney tumor was discovered accidently, as he had no symptoms, swelling, or weight gain. Initially he was told it had spread to his liver, though it was ultimately and fortunately found that there was no metastasis to any other organs. The surgery to remove the tumor was delicate and a medical team of different specialties was assembled for the five-plus hour operation. David and his family were told he might not survive the surgery, but his being in excellent physical shape may have made the difference. The tumor weighed in at twelve pounds if you can believe that. David lost a kidney, but is doing fine today.*

> *Harvey has had multiple cancers over the past eleven years as have many family members. Though he has difficulties walking and needs two canes or a motorized scooter, he is doing well, and still pursues his passion of traveling around the world with his wife Carol.*

> *My friend Rosemary had colon cancer in 2012. The robot surgery perforated her colon causing multiple complications, re-hospitalizations, and a lingering infection for six months. At one point she was not allowed to eat solid food for more than a month. Now she is fine and back to living and enjoying her life. She and her husband just enjoyed a ten-day cruise, and she looks and feels wonderful.*

To live in hearts we leave behind is not to die.

—Clyde Campbell

Time flies whether you are having fun or not so you better have some fun.

—William Penzer, Ph.D.

Time goes, you say? Ah no! Alas, time stays, we go.

—Henry Dobson

Yesterday is a cancelled check: Forget it. Tomorrow is a promissory not: Don't count on it. Today is ready cash. Use it.

—Edwin Bliss

I have an intention to live each day's moments, fully.

—Valerie Harper
Diagnosed with incurable brain cancer

Life is for the living. Death is for the dead. Let life be like music. And death a note unsaid.

—*Langston Hughes*

I used to want the words "She tried," on my tombstone. Now I want, "She did it."

—*Katherine Dunham*

Count reminiscences like money.

—*Carl Sandburg*

Here is a test to find whether your mission on Earth is finished; if you're alive, it isn't.

—*Richard Bach*

There are so many more stories than these, so please see them as both symbolic and inspiring. But here comes my tight rope dance—I sadly know that not everyone makes in through the Cancerville maze. But I sincerely hope that you will, and let's just assume that will be the case.

I want to share another story that might offer a service that can help anyone wanting to leave a legacy. Todd's mom died of cancer when he was an infant. There were a few pictures that he saw of her when he was young, but not much else. When he was an adult, an uncle gave him a box of memorabilia that included a letter Todd's mom wrote to her brother and sister-in-law, thanking them for taking care of Todd when she was in a cancer center far from home. Seeing his mom's handwriting triggered a strong surge of emotion, which ultimately let to creating ZarpZ.com with his friend Diptesh. They are both pharmaceutical researchers and little surprise that Todd specializes in discovering new drugs for cancer.

To accomplish their goal they together invested more than one hundred thousand dollars to have ZarpZ.com built. As you will see it is a legacy website where pictures, videos, notes, cards, etc. can be uploaded and sent via email to anyone at a specified date. I can leave birthday wishes, graduation congrats to my new granddaughter, a love note to my wife, etc. to be delivered after I pass on. So can you, if you so choose. There is no charge for this service.

To me, it is very interesting that Todd's mom had such a strong influence on him, even though she passed before he got to know her or she him. In this story, there is much inspiration too. We just never know the power of our legacies, and the interesting ways we can have an impact long after we are gone.

Experts agree that it is important for us to learn about our options, talk about our preferences, prepare directives in advance, inform our loved ones and doctors about our desires, document everything, and of course, chill the Cristal at just the right temperature. I can do all of that and assume you can too!

Remember, you are not only a cancer patient, **YOU ARE A SURVIVOR!** Live your life fully, try to enjoy every day, even the difficult ones, kick some ass while yours is being kicked in Cancerville, heal physically and emotionally, and believe with all your heart and soul that this too will pass and you will not! Assume that your life will continue on, having learned some valuable life lessons from your Cancerville experiences (see Chapter 24 *How to Cope Better When You Have Cancer*). Hair grows back, minds come back, and lives come back too. Enjoy yours for as long as you have here on Earth. Being born is a privilege, living is too, and dying, well that's just the price of admission.

I know it is coming (his death), and I don't fear it, because I believe there is nothing on the other side of death to fear…. I was perfectly content before I was born, and I think of death as the same state. I am grateful for the gifts of intelligence, love, wonder and laughter.
—Roger Ebert
    Film Critic

Activity 1:

Circle all of the planning actions you have taken for whenever you move on to take your rightful place in Heaven:

- Consulted a lawyer
- Created a will and estate plan
- Have a clear health care directive
- Looked into a "Physician's Orders for Life-Sustaining Treatment" (POLST)
- Created powers of attorney
- Assigned a person to make health care decisions if you are not able
- Made all funeral/cremation arrangements ahead of time
- Left clear instructions as to your wishes after you pass on
- Left a legacy at ZarpZ.com for future delivery
- Bought that bottle of Cristal and resisted the temptation to drink it all!

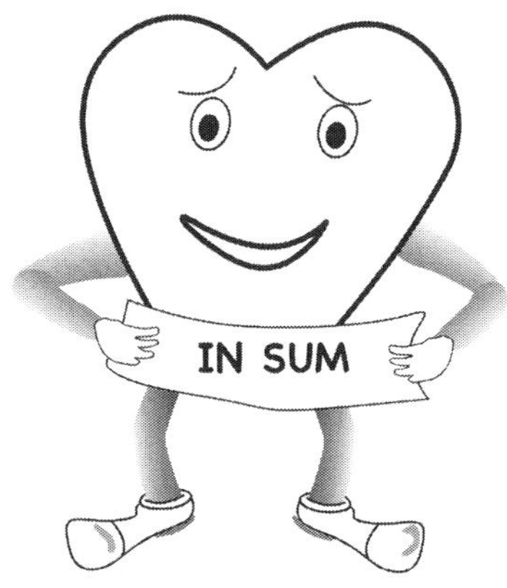

CHAPTER 22

Summarization

I hope I have helped you find strength, while riding through Cancerville on a horse I call Hope. My goal has been to provide you with a variety of actions that conspire to inspire you in "DAM STRONG!" directions. It has also been to reach out to you with my words in a warm and heartfelt way.

I tried my best to write this book as if we were sitting across from one another in my backyard on a bright sunny day. In addition, I strived to be real, honest, and open, doing my best to acknowledge the harsh realities of Cancerville, while balancing those against my encouragements. I wanted to be realistic, rather than naïve and idealistic. I also tried to provide you with a series of activities that enabled you to take charge of "mission control" in Cancerville, as well as become even more "DAM STRONG!"

Obviously, much will depend upon your unique and personal situation and experience. Some of my encouragements will fit snugly, while others may not be appropriate. Many of the general principles, however, will be relevant across the board:

- Dam grams of pride bank deposits trump shame and blame every day of the week, though we all can be "weak" at times.
- Optimism rules the day, but pessimisms can creep into the strongest of us.
- Hope springs eternal, of that there is no doubt, but Cancerville challenges our hope generator regularly, and can throw us forcefully off the Hope horse.
- The need for social support in Cancerville is undeniable, but so is one's sense of aloneness, even when surrounded by family and friends.
- Staying organized is helpful, but Cancerville overwhelms the most together of people, and causes them to throw their hands and their papers in the air.
- Truth be known we are all in a footrace with our destiny, but Cancerville underscores the thin ice upon which we all tread.
- The tools offered throughout the Workbook are intended to support your journey, and help you get past all of these speed bumps quickly.

As I read the above bullets I just typed, I realized that Cancerville is a high wire balancing act. You will have your good days and your off days; you will laugh and you will cry. At times, you may do both on the same

Idealism increases in direct proportion to one's distance from the problem.

—Unknown

All human wisdom is summed up in two words—wait and hope.

—Alexander Dumas

The art of the quoter is to know when to stop.

—Robertson Davies

day, or even within the same hour. Both are necessary and healthy vents. At times, you will feel strong and at other times you will feel weakened, as if by kryptonite. That said, I am hopeful and confident that you will return to your superman/superwoman strength as quickly as possible.

Clearly having cancer sucks—there's no denying that fact. Unfortunately, most unfortunately, that is the hand you were dealt. I am sincerely sad and sorry that your life has been so burdened. But surviving cancer does not suck. That too is an undeniable truth. Remember that **You are Not Only a Cancer Patient You are a SURVIVOR!** Your challenge is to play a poor hand well, and I am optimistic you are doing just that everyday.

Toward the goal I wish you well.

Don't ignore what you feel—it can help to express your emotions. Mourn your losses. They are real, and you have a right to grieve. Then, try to focus on the ways that coping with cancer has made you stronger, wiser, and more realistic. There is so much that makes you valuable.
—Young Survival Coalition

Printed in Dunstable, United Kingdom